the pregnancy quiz
Try the quiz at the start of your pregnancy and then again at the end, and see how far you've come.

1 Colostrum is:
a) a very attractive ruin near the Colosseum
b) stuff that comes out of your boobs when you start to breastfeed
c) that strange goo that newborn babies are covered in
d) a thrash-trance band from near Seattle

2 Can you retain fluid and be dehydrated at the same time?
a) don't be ridiculous
b) oh, God, yes
c) it depends on what star sign you are

3 Should you try to get time off before the baby arrives, rather than work until the due date?
a) yes
b) uh-huh
c) ooh, yeah
d) damn straight

4 Which is the most relaxing birth support team?
a) a midwife and your partner, sister, or friend
b) a film crew; a live-on-the-Internet technical support team; a still photographer; your children, parents, and second cousins; all the girls from work; and somebody called Arthur who took a wrong turn on the way to the cafeteria
c) nobody at all

5 Inducement is:
a) a very large diamond ring and a vacation in the Bahamas
b) an artificial medical process to stimulate labor
c) holding a Milk Dud at the end of the vagina to coax the baby out
d) a technical term for the placement of the placenta

▶

6 Braxton Hicks is:

a) that lantern-jawed guy who slept with his aunt on *The Bold and the Beautiful*

b) a term coined by NASA astronauts for a false alarm, named after an over-excited engineer on the Apollo 12 mission

c) prelabor contractions

d) a combination of the two most popular baby names in Kentucky in 1897

7 Palpation is:

a) what happens to your cervix when you have an orgasm

b) a pretentious word for "copping a feel"

c) the medical term for the faster heart rate you attain toward the end of a pregnancy

d) the opposite of temptation or craving: something that makes you nauseated

8 Placenta is:

a) the most popular girls' name after Sarah, Rebecca, and Madison

b) the geographical location where you have your baby

c) a big gloopy item that looks like a liver and keeps the fetus alive with nutrients and oxygen

d) a terrific marketing opportunity if you put it through a blender, add it to a moisturizer, and give it a French name

9 The easiest way of giving birth is by:

a) taking all the drugs you can get your hands on and shouting a lot at random

b) imagining you're in a perfectly charming wheat field having sex with George Clooney

c) having a general anesthetic and paying someone to look after the baby for the first ten years

d) by whatever means are necessary at the time

e) copying what they do in the movies

10 **Women who say childbirth doesn't really hurt are:**
a) lucky
b) deluded
c) insane
d) men

11 **A primigravida is:**
a) one of those ballerinas who don't eat enough
b) a woman giving birth for the first time
c) the first time you feel the baby move inside you

12 **Living with a newborn baby is:**
a) just like a lovely vacation
b) exhausting
c) what was the question again?

13 **If you don't have a husband, you can:**
a) get help from relatives and friends
b) just go straight to hell, you floozy Miss Jezebel person
c) claim benefits through the welfare program

14 **Postpartum means after the birth. Antenatal means:**
a) prenatal, or before the birth
b) you're against the whole idea of pregnancy, or being in any way natal
c) another word for childbirth

15 **Sex is:**
a) really a tremendously heightened sensual experience all through pregnancy
b) just asking for trouble
c) apparently something that single, childless people do in their spare time ■

MRS. FANNY BRAXTON HICKS

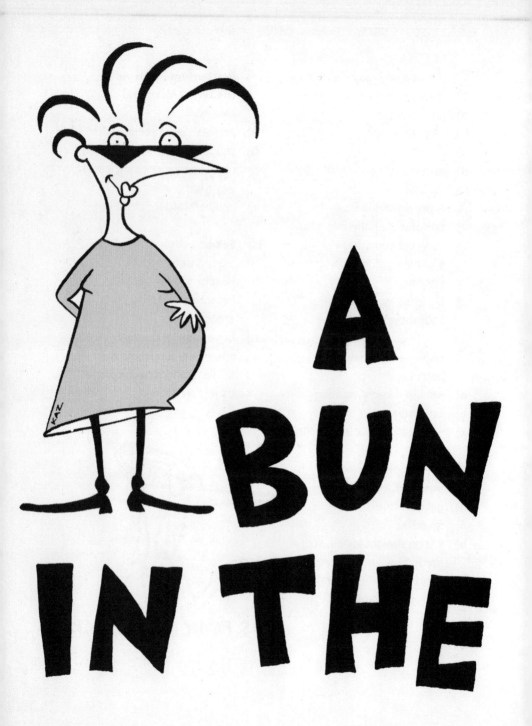

KAZ COOKE

The **real guide to pregnancy**

OVEN

TEN SPEED PRESS
Berkeley | Toronto

Ten Speed Press
P.O. Box 7123
Berkeley, California 94707
www.tenspeed.com

Originally published in 1999 by Penguin Books Australia.

Designed by Sandy Cull and Leonie Atott
Production work for U.S. edition by Betsy Stromberg

Library of Congress Cataloging-in-Publication Data on file the publisher.
ISBN 1-58008-531-8

Printed in Canada
First printing, 2003

1 2 3 4 5 6 7 8 9 10 — 08 07 06 05 04 03

for Oofty Goofty

contents

"VERTICAL STRIPES FLATTER THE MATERNAL FIGURE" — SALES ASSISTANT

Intro

Why did I write this book? Aren't there enough pregnancy gurus? For a start the last thing you need when you're pregnant is a bossy-boots insisting you "should" feel this and "must" do that. Who wants to have, or be, a guru? Not me. OK, so first, I realized I had a bun in the oven. Then realized I had no idea what I was in for.

I bought a squillion pregnancy books and discovered they often contradict each other on key points; or they're written by rich women who think you should get a sink installed in your child's bedroom (I ask you) or by people pushing their own personal theory, which may or may not involve giving birth in a wading pool full of lavender water and the dog.

The other thing pregnancy books tend to do is describe the size of the developing fetus in comparison with food. One week it's a Brazil nut, then a plum, then an eggplant. At one point I became convinced I was going to give birth to a giant muesli.

And most of the books finish at exactly week 40, when the baby is due. In real life, while you're pregnant, you can't think any farther than the birth. But the very minute you have a baby you can hardly remember a thing about the pregnancy. It's suddenly entirely irrelevant and you have to deal IMMEDIATELY with a tiny person who depends on you completely (and also do stuff with your boobs they don't even ask of exotic dancers).

For some reason I had always imagined that being pregnant would just be like being me but with a big bump out the front. It hadn't occurred to me that the reality of being pregnant eventually would be felt constantly in every physical part of my body, and in every recess of what I used to fondly call my mind. Even though I had heard about nausea and fluid retention and vagueness and a ferzillion other things, for some dumb reason I thought they were part of an old-fashioned pregnancy, relegated to history along with the concept of "confinement" and Mrs. Spinoza's mechanical home-perm-and-gherkin-bottling machine.

I'm a career woman, I thought. I'm over 30. I've always pretended to be in control of my life, and that doesn't have to stop just because I'm pregnant. I'll just live my life the way it has always been (without getting drunk and having a few cigarettes on the weekend). Work will go on as normal and life at home will be just the same, only I'll need bigger shirts at some point. My life will only completely change once the baby comes out.

WELL.

Apparently not.

I had not bargained on the body taking control of itself. The power of the mind? Pah, and furthermore, snorty snonking sound. As far as my body was concerned, its major priority was growing a healthy baby. Several times I felt my legs going off along the hall for a nap when I thought my torso should have been elsewhere. I woke up in the middle of the night feeling compelled to eat banana sandwiches and drink glasses of soy milk. I had become a host organ.

My first thoughts every morning and my last thoughts at night were about being pregnant, and there was a fair amount of it in between. (This is as well as the other stuff you usually have to be on top of in your normal life.) Would I be a good mother? What if something went wrong? Was it too late to have second thoughts? Should I feel guilty about having second thoughts? Where do we stand on third and subsequent thoughts? Where the hell are my keys? Why is the peanut butter in the freezer? Did I do that? What the hell has happened to my HAIR? What's that weird bump forming on my gums? Do stretch marks stay that lovely shade of royal purple forever? Will I ever want to have sex again? What do people mean when they say "pregnancy hormones"? Is it true some aromatherapy can make me have a miscarriage? Is it any wonder they keep making horror movies about motherhood and the creatures inside us? Isn't this miraculous? Isn't this uncomfortable? Isn't this terrifying, and wonderful, and fascinating, and boring as batshit, all at the same time? Am I supposed to feel serene, or just seasick? If I don't do my pelvic-floor exercises will my vagina fall out? Why can't I feel the baby move yet? Could the baby stop moving for a while and give me a rest? What about those cigarettes I had before I realized I was pregnant? Will I ever be able to be alone again? How can I tell people I don't want my career back? How can I get my career back? When does a fetus become a baby? Does that mean if it's born then it will survive? Could I get any fatter? What's preeclampsia and how do you get it? What can you see on an ultrasound screen? What if labor goes on forever and nothing comes out? Could somebody get me a cup of tea?

And then when I had a baby the questions *really* started.

So to find out what's what, I wrote *A Bun in the Oven*. The researchers and I went to work, and then experts checked everything written about their special area and suggested new bits, and then the editor asked a gadzillion questions, and in the normal course of events I would have had a huge tantrum but I was too tired because by that time I'd had a baby, so instead we checked it all over again and took bits out and put bits in and waved it all about, and now here it is.

If you read everything in the book you might think pregnancy is a terrible minefield of bizarre health complaints. Don't freak out: lots of the pregnancy problems are rare—they're included just in case. If you do have a special interest or problem, though, this book will give you the basics. And if there's something you need to know more about, you can find an organization or book that will point you in the right direction recommended in the Help section (that's the bit toward the end).

— Kaz

P.S.: Oh, yeah. The Diary of Maddie the Modern Girl's pregnancy includes many aspects of my own experience, with a few stories from other people thrown in and the odd embellishment. It is not quite my story. A girl has to try to cling to some sense of mystery (especially when she's got baby vomit up her nose). (Don't ask.)

TeRmS of ENdeARMeNt

From conception we call the developing baby an EMBRYO, even in its earliest, cell-dividing days. At 10 weeks, the embryo becomes a FETUS, although you'll find that the term is often used for the unborn baby at all stages from conception to birth. All its organ systems are formed by then, and it's ready to expend most of its energy on maturing and growing.

At 28 weeks the fetus becomes a BABY, even though a lot of medical staff still call it a fetus right up until it's born. We've called it a baby from week 28 because many premature babies born at this stage are likely to survive with modern hospital care.

PREGNANCY SPEAK

The trimesters
Trimester means three months, so:

⊚ The first trimester is up to the end of week 13.

⊚ The second trimester is week 14 to the end of week 26.

⊚ The third trimester is week 27 until birth.

Dates
This book, like most doctors, counts your pregnancy from the first day of your last period. So even if technically you conceived two weeks ago, you're 4 weeks pregnant.

what's going on

Not much. By the end of the week, you've just finished the last period you'll have for a while. You're into the follicular phase of the menstrual cycle, which means the egg-making and dispatch phase (follicle is the name for the tiny sac in which the egg matures). One of your two ovaries is deciding which of the eggs developing in this menstrual cycle will be the one to go forth. (An egg is also known as an ovum, if you want to get all Latin about it.) Your ovaries release 400–500 mature eggs during your "fertile" years. It only takes one to get pregnant.

Your body is going about its usual hormonal carry-on. Lots of estrogen (actually several estrogens, just called "estrogen" as an umbrella term) is being produced by your ovaries. This stimulates the uterus to grow more lining, called the endometrium, to replace the lining that has just left as your last period. This new endometrium is the welcoming surface for the egg if it's fertilized. The egg is extremely teeny: about the size of the head of a straight pin.

DIARY I took an inventory of my life recently and wrote it down with an eyebrow pencil on the back of a brown paper bag that used to have a muffin in it. It pretty much came out this way:

✳ Madeline Harridan.

✳ Age: 32.

✳ Unglamorous fashion designer for small struggling rag trade company, Real Gorgeous Pty. Ltd. (we make the Real Women Wear label, sizes 4–14).

✳ Sagittarius (tactless and jovial).

✳ Hobbies: eating, sleeping, buying shoes.

✳ Accoutrements: perfectly decent boyfriend called Matt, who works in a garden shop. Part of a house, mortgaged. Nice couch. $3,500 in the bank.

✳ Shape: not unlike the fruit known colloquially as a pear. With legs. Unusually fat knees. Never mind. Rest of self reasonably overweight, but nothing that a lot of exercise and a little less reliance on chocolate and cheese wouldn't cure.

✳ Medical history: long tussle with endometriosis, a menstrual condition that often causes infertility, which I have controlled by taking the Pill full-time without a break. Haven't had a period for four years.

✳ Doctor's advice last time I went: if you want to get pregnant, come off the Pill and start boinking like a rabbit (or words to that effect).

So Matt and I had a talk. Six months before, I'd said I wanted to have kids and he'd said it was too soon (he's only 31, my toyboy). This time, though, he'd thought about it and was as ready as he'd ever be, particularly since I told him that, given my medical history, nothing at all might happen, or it might take two years to get everything working again. I told Matt there were a few things to sort out: Like what would we do if a test during pregnancy showed that the baby had Down's Syndrome? And how would he feel if the kid grew up to be a gay man?

Matt put his head to the side and thought for a moment, "As long as he roots for the Giants I can't see the problem."

We each made a list of stuff we'd have to do before I got pregnant. Mine said:

∗ Go off Pill, and see Beck (that's my herbalist and medical adviser and fellow champagne admirer) about what else I should be on instead.

∗ Lose weight.

∗ Get fit.

∗ Buy lottery ticket.

∗ Stop smoking.

∗ Stop drinking.

∗ Get driver's license.

∗ Don't roll about in pesticide-soaked fields, stop eating junk food, cook magnificently cunning little low-fat dishes from primary food sources, stop saying "fuck" so much, get legs waxed, organize the sanding of the floor of our new house without actually breathing in any of that polyurethane topcoat. (The sanders, who breathe it in all day long, seem to have the IQ of somebody called Igor in a lab coat.)

I duct-taped the list of things to do onto the fridge. Then I took it off and replaced it with a note on a small piece of the muffin bag saying, "Change entire life immediately," and threw my packet of Pills in the trash in a melodramatic fashion.

There was absolutely nothing on Matt's list except:

∗ Buy milk and bread.

∗ Have sex.

info

getting ready for pregnancy

This is the time—before you get pregnant—to tackle any relationship problems or sort out any mixed feelings you have about life and pregnancy. Why do you want to have a baby? Do you want a toddler and a teenager? (That's what babies become.) Have you talked it all out with your partner, if you have one? Will the father be involved after the baby is born? How can you protect yourself from sexually transmitted diseases while trying to get pregnant? Is pregnancy going to spoil your chances of getting that part in *Bikini Busters: The Sequel*?

Some people think that having a baby will bring them closer together. These people should take a pill and lie down. Having a baby is probably the most stressful thing you'll ever do. Everyone quotes Nora Ephron: "A baby is a hand grenade thrown into a marriage." And there's all the practical stuff to think about *before* you have a bun in the oven:

⑥ Are you really ready to make the transition from ready-for-anything-at-a-moment's-notice to slave-to-baby-Mommy-who-hasn't-had-time-to-shower-in-two-days-and-whose-every-outing-must-be-planned-with-a-military-precision-that-needs-to-be-totally-flexible-if-the-baby-wakes-up/won't-wake-up/cries/vomits/ needs-feeding/poops-on-the-cell-phone? If you postpone the decision, does that mean you might later be trying to get pregnant when your fertility is declining rapidly?

⑥ If you have a partner, this is a very fine time to share your ideas about parenting, to avoid heartache farther down the track. Do you need to move in together? Are you both going to stop smoking? What are your views on prenatal (also referred to as "antenatal") testing? What would you do if you found out your child had a severe abnormality or a disabling condition? How would you cope with the idea of terminating the pregnancy, or living with a baby who would grow up always having special needs? Will the baby be part of a religious group? If it's a boy, will you have him circumcised? (Many of these issues are explored in this book and you can look up topics such as prenatal testing and circumcision in the Index.)

⑥ What child-care arrangements do you see as ideal? What's going to be possible, or affordable? How about education? Who does most of the housework and other unpaid jobs around the house, and would that need to change? Do you share the same feelings about the possibility of your child growing up to be gay, or a stockbroker? What are your views on discipline and the issue of spanking children? Do you have a good support network of family and friends? Have any of them had recent experience with babies? Do you have an alternate plan for any of this stuff?

⑥ Do you need to take out health insurance? If you want private obstetric and hospital care and to be able to choose your own obstetrician, you do need insurance, and you need to get it *before* you get pregnant. Make sure you check exactly what they'll pay for. Many only cover some in-hospital expenses, and no out-of-hospital bills.

⑥ See your health care provider and naturopath and announce that you've decided you're going to try to get pregnant. They can give you a clean bill of health to start with, and they will probably recommend that you start taking a special pre-pregnancy multivitamin supplement that includes zinc and folate and excludes vitamin A, which can harm an unborn baby. Folate, or folic acid, can reduce your risk of having a baby with spina bifida or a related problem. You need to *start* taking a vitamin with 8 mg (800 mcg) of folic acid for at least three months before conception. As you would with any supplements, check with your doctor that folate is compatible with any other drugs you are taking. (See Eating and Supplements in Week 2 for more info on zinc and folate.)

◉ If you don't have immunity to it, get vaccinated against rubella (German measles), which can harm an unborn baby. Be careful not to conceive until three months after the shot. You may also need new vaccinations or booster shots for diseases such as tetanus or hepatitis B. (And if you think you could already be pregnant, check with your doctor about vaccinations, as some can cause damage to an unborn baby.)

◉ If you suffer from a chronic health problem (for example, asthma, heart disease, liver problems, thyroid disease, diabetes, epilepsy, multiple sclerosis, or mental illness), you should discuss medications and the management of your condition during pregnancy with your health care provider or a perinatologist (high-risk pregnancy specialist) before you conceive.

◉ If you or your partner has a family history of hereditary disorders, speak to your doctor about seeing a genetic counselor before conceiving (see Genetic Counseling in Week 10). If either you or your partner have Jewish ancestry, get tested for Tay-Sachs disease. Tay-Sachs disease occurs more frequently in people with Jewish heritage. If either you or your partner are African American, a test for sickle-cell anemia should be done. Caucasians should be tested for cystic fibrosis. A regular blood count can be done to screen for thalassemia if either you or your partner have Mediterranean descent. These conditions are rare, even in the "high-risk" ethnic groups.

◉ Planned Parenthood clinics (see Family Planning Clinics in Help), like your doctor, can advise you on all sorts of things, from termination to where to get support throughout your pregnancy, at the birth, and afterward.

⊚ The fitter and healthier you are going into conception and pregnancy, the better. Growing another human being is a huge workload and it's a job that goes on twenty-four hours a day for about nine months. If you're trying to get pregnant, the following are important: eat healthy food and take your prenatal vitamins after consulting your doctor (see Eating and Supplements in Week 2); exercise; stop smoking, drinking, and taking recreational drugs (see Looking After Your Embryo and Fetus in Week 4); tell your doctor or pharmacist you might be pregnant before you buy prescription or over-the-counter medications or herbal treatments; and aim to increase or decrease your weight so that it's within the recommended range for your height and build. (This is not the weight your Aunt Verna or *Cosmopolitan* magazine thinks you should be. It's called the Body Mass Index calculation and it's only relevant if you're over 18 and completely finished growing. Ask your doctor about it.) Some hospitals have special programs for overweight or underweight women to increase their fertility (see Hospitals in Help for phone numbers).

⊚ If you have a male partner, encourage him to adopt a healthy diet and lifestyle so he will be producing healthy sperm when you conceive (in other words, try not to have unprotected sex with a drug fiend who won't eat his greens).

⊚ Go to the dentist. You may as well get any dental work that includes X-rays, anesthetics, or medication out of the way before conception rather than having to wait until after the birth.

⊚ If you are over 40, be sure your mammograms are up to date. Once you are pregnant and while breastfeeding, you will not be able to have a mammogram.

⊚ Check out your rights to parental leave with your employer. In a large company you may be able to do this anonymously by phone if you don't want to flag your intentions. And check your rights with your union or the relevant government department, as well as your employer. The Family and Medical Leave Act (FMLA) states that most employers must grant an eligible employee up to twelve weeks of unpaid leave. In most states, women are also eligible for short-term disability to pay for a portion or all of their maternity leave. Some employers offer other benefits worth pursuing, including flexible working arrangements after the baby is born, and work-based child care. If there are two working parents involved, find out whose job offers a better package and child-care arrangements. If you're on contract or a temporary employee, you may not have any rights.

◎ If one parent is taking time off paid work to look after the baby, how are your family finances going to be reorganized? (How do you spell "budget"?) How would you feel about a joint account? Or about an automatic transferral of money from the income of the paid partner to the account of the one at home with the baby? Do you need to start a special savings account in case of emergencies? Would it be a good idea to rob a bank at this point?

◎ If you plan to renovate your house, arrange to have jobs that could be harmful to the pregnancy—such as stripping old, lead-based paint or sealing sanded floorboards with polyurethane—carried out before you conceive, or stay somewhere else while they are being done.

◎ Make sure items around the house are environmentally friendly and avoid fumes or other fetus-threatening situations: have gas heaters, microwave ovens, and other appliances checked and serviced to make sure they're not leaking carbon monoxide, radiation, or anything else a bit spooky.

◎ If you're buying a car, make sure it has an anchor point for a baby seat. Most cars built after August 1, 2002 will have the anchor point; most built before that date won't. If you have an older car, you'll need to use the car's seat belts to strap in the child seat.

◎ Buy a lottery ticket. If you win, buy a great washing machine, a dryer, a new fridge, and a cordless phone you can carry from

SPECIAL HINTS FROM A MOTHER
Before you decide to have a baby:
- spend time with friends who already have a baby, or older children, and have a good, hard look at their life.
- spend at least a full day from dawn until late with a mother and a small baby; it's impossible to imagine just how much work is involved until you are in the thick of it.

room to room that has a hands-free speaker function. If your house doesn't have good heating or cooling and you need it in your climate, install it. Book a fully qualified nanny through a reputable nanny agency to come and help you in the first couple of weeks at home. If there's any money left over, get yourself a vacation and an emerald tiara.

trying to get pregnant

If you're trying to get pregnant, make absolutely sure you know which times of the month are most fertile for you: probably about day 14 if you have a 28 day cycle, counting the first day of your last period as day 1. Your doctor can help you with discussions about ovulation, fertile mucus, and the other nitty-gritties.

According to in vitro specialist Professor David de Kretzer, you shouldn't keep trying forever. If you're not pregnant after a year of having unprotected sex, get a referral from your local doctor to a medical fertility specialist. If you're approaching 40, don't leave it as long as a year. Generally speaking, your fertility declines steadily after 35 and plunges after 40.

It may be a good idea to see someone even before you start trying. An obstetrician or fertility expert can talk to you about ways to maximize your chances of conception based on your individual situation. (Conception rates for your age group, for example, could be irrelevant to you if you have a medical condition that's preventing conception.)

If you're having trouble, see Infertility in Help, as well as your doctor.

BOOKS FOR PRE-PREGNANCY

 Healthy Parents, Better Babies: A Couple's Guide to Natural Preconception Health Care by Francesca Naish and Janette Roberts, Crossing Press, Berkeley, CA.
Offers natural ways and various theories to improve your health and fitness before getting pregnant. It also aims to improve fertility, but of course this will not work for everyone.

Planning a Baby: How to Prepare for a Healthy Pregnancy and Give Your Baby the Best Possible Start by Dr. Sarah Brewer, Optima, London, 1996.

A medical perspective from England, including sections on vitamins, exercise, sexually transmitted diseases, male sexual health, trying to conceive, and miscarriage.

REALITY CHICKS

The Mask of Motherhood: How Mothering Changes Everything and Why We Pretend It Doesn't by Susan Maushart, Penguin, New York, 2000.

The author is a social scientist who talks about the possible negatives of mothering, including the loss of a sense of self, the breastfeeding propaganda war, the chaos and confusion, the pain, the lot. She reminds us that for every woman who says breastfeeding is a wildly erotic and bonding experience, there are others who feel like a milking cow limping from one disaster to the next. And that for every model looking radiant in a magazine with a clean, new baby, there are other women madly trying to juggle offspring, work, a house, and relationships.

Life after Birth: What Even Your Friends Won't Tell You about Motherhood by Kate Figes, St. Martin's Press, New York, 2002.

This book is actually about the unglamorous side of things. The list of contents tells the story, including "Childbirth: Just the Beginning," "Emotions," "Exhaustion," "Relations with the Father," "Friends and the Outside World." Resources are all relevant to England, not the United States.

Read any of the books about how to care for a baby (see Baby-Care Books in Week 43). It will give you a tiny inkling of what you're in for.

your record

Write down your thoughts here and in the other
Your Record sections of the book, so that in the
future you can look back at your pregnancy and recall
your experience.

The changes you made to get ready for pregnancy:

Why do you want to have a baby?

What do you imagine looking after a baby
will be like?

How do you think your life will change after the
baby? What do you think you will do about working
outside the home?

what's going on

By about day 14 (day 1 is the first day of your last period), you've reached the dispatch stage and your body is ready to ovulate. This means this month's dominant egg is released from one of your ovaries and waved into the nearby opening of a fallopian tube by tentacly-looking bits on the end of the tube. You have two fallopian tubes, one on each side of the uterus, providing the link between each ovary and the uterus. At the time of ovulation, your vaginal mucous (look, you're going to hear a lot worse words and concepts than vaginal mucous in the next nine months so pull yourself together) usually looks like raw egg whites and is known as "fertile mucous" and at some point you'll have to get some sperm up there. Most women do this by having sex with a guy: this is still the easiest method.

After this week, you'll be into the "proliferative" part of your menstrual cycle. This means the endometrium (the lining of the uterus) is "proliferating"—growing like mad.

Diary I decide to blow our savings and take Matt away to Hawaii for a week to ravish him constantly. Before we go I see my herbalist, Beck, who's also had years of experience as a hospital midwife.

She gives me a tonic and some vitamins that include something called folate and heaven knows what other baby-friendly stuff, in preparation for Operation Bun in the Oven. Matt and I both need a vacation to fortify us anyway, having been working like demons to pay for the new house.

I believe there are many ways you can pinpoint the moment of ovulation, involving thermometers, ropes and pulleys, and other implements. I should have got out the calculator and a protractor and a slide rule and a sextant and a sexton and half a sundial to work out when I might ovulate. (Don't know what a sexton is, but it sounds raunchy.) I haven't enough endometrium to have a period, but that's how it is when you come off the Pill after four years on it nonstop. A menstrual chart's about as much use to me as a stuffed aardvark.

Instead I just guess.

So ten days after I've come off the Pill, I am poised for Operation Ravishment. Matt keeps looking up from his beach towel and science fiction novel and saying, "Hello, is it that time again?" when he sees the look in my eye, and manfully trailing me back to the hut. But in between ravishings and drinking champagne, I start to have second thoughts about being pregnant.

This could be a big year for me at work, even the chance of designing my own small range of clothes. I'm in line for promotion to head designer of Real Women Wear (stuff sold to people you or I might know, in things called "shops," as opposed to what's known rather unkindly in the industry as "Sluts on Stilts Wear": the flashier end of the collections called "couture," the mad, show-offy bits that end up only on catwalk models).

I go over and over the decision, obsessing about all the things I couldn't have if I had a baby: independence, a disposable income, velvet shoes, the chance of being able to walk out the door and catch a plane or go shopping by myself, vomit-free shoulders, boobs I can call my own. And I know women whose partners say they'll "help" instead of "I'll do half" and house husbands (primary caregivers, thank you very much) who play with the kids but don't cook the dinner or do any cleaning.

I keep double-checking with Matt that he really wants to stay home the first year of the baby's life while I go out to work, and that he'll also do the cleaning. Then I start panicking—as I'm sure most guys do—that I've got to bring home the bacon and stay employed for the next twenty years. We have long conversations about changing my mind, what it will do to my career, how being childless would be so much easier.

After a particularly well-executed ravishing on Tuesday morning I lie there looking at the languid ceiling fan with the definite feeling that *that* was exactly the sort of behavior that would get one pregnant, if one were able to get pregnant. Which of course triggers the decision to go back on the Pill as soon as I get home and postpone the whole thing.

"It's all right, Madeline," according to Matt the Ravishee. "Plenty of time. It's up to you."

Then he says something terribly sensible, which is that there is never an ideal time to have a baby unless you're the sort of person who has nothing to do all day, gobs of money, and a spare teddy bear. Neither of us falls into this category, but really it could be worse. We're both employed, we've got somewhere to live and a car, and neither of us has a conviction for aggravated assault. And even if things were not so good, we'd work it out somehow. Still, it might be better to just wait and see if I get the promotion before I spend any more energy swinging from the chandelier in the nude making diverting remarks about likely ovulation days. Metaphorically speaking.

info

eating and supplements

You usually need more than the standard requirements of energy, protein, and certain vitamins and minerals when you're pregnant, although you might be getting nearly everything you need already (and no, a whiskey and a stack of pancakes each day does not keep the doctor away).

Basically, you've got to pay attention to your overall intake of everything to sustain the healthy growth and development of your baby. Not to mention getting through pregnancy without fainting around the joint and being all gaunt and frazzled.

How many calories you need will depend on your age, height, build, weight at the time of conception, current diet, and whether you're a couch potato. Remember that for almost everyone it's important to put on weight during pregnancy. This is no time to go on a weight-loss diet or a fast. Either could be very dangerous for your baby and you.

The average recommended increase is 300 calories a day. You need to add more than this if you were underweight to start with, if you're a teenager, or if you're carrying more than one baby. Your individual diet should be discussed with your midwife, naturopath, doctor, obstetrician, or pregnancy dietician.

To keep your weight gain within recommended limits while giving your baby all the goodies it needs, and so you don't get madly hungry, you need to eat quality calories. Fresh, seasonal food provides far more nutrients than highly processed convenience and junk foods.

Most people can get all the nutrients, vitamins, and minerals necessary for a healthy pregnancy from a well-planned, balanced, and varied diet. And the vitamins and nutrients you eat are always better in value than ones in tablets or capsules.

But who always eats a perfectly balanced diet? No one unless they've got a private chef and time, dedication, and squillions of dollars. You could be frantically busy and not quite eating what you should. Or throwing up could be leaving you depleted of vital nutrients. Or you might be trying to get through pregnancy on a vegan diet (no animal products), which is just not adequate for fetal development. (You may want to reconsider your vegan status during your pregnancy.) Special recommendations for vegans and vegetarians are scattered throughout this section.

Taking some supplements during pregnancy can be a good way of improving your intake of nutrients if your diet isn't perfect. Remember to talk to your doctor before taking any supplements prescribed for you by somebody else or that you've bought independently. (Early routine blood tests can identify pre-existing deficiencies in iron, vitamin B12, and folate.)

Your individual needs for certain supplements and doses will be different from those of anyone else, so talk about them with your dietician, midwife, doctor, obstetrician, or naturopath. Some multivitamin supplements (BUT NOT ALL, especially ones with vitamin A added) are fine and dandy during pregnancy because they combine a lot of your needs in one pill, but read all labels carefully.

warning: vitamin A

Excessive levels of vitamin A are associated with birth defects, including cleft palate and heart malformation. Don't take any vitamin A supplement while pregnant, outside of your prenatal vitamins. Sometimes vitamin A turns up in unexpected places such as a B-group vitamin supplement. Avoid eating pâté or liver (which is full of vitamin A and may be full of chemicals, such as cadmium).

protein

You'll usually need an extra 25 grams a day on top of your non-pregnant requirement. That means you need a total of 5 to 6 servings of protein a day: 1 serving could be 1 glass of low-fat milk (unless you need the fat); 1 ounce of hard cheese; 5 ounces of yogurt; 3¹/₂ ounces of lean meat; 7 ounces of fish; or 1 cup of cooked beans or lentils.

Vegetarians need to be really strict about combining grains with legumes—to maximize the quality of their protein intake. Protein-rich foods include miso, tofu, eggs, dairy foods, seaweeds, nuts, and seeds. Vegans will need to pay special attention to their protein requirements.

If you've been vegetarian or vegan and crave meat while you're pregnant, listen to your body and eat meat or fish if it doesn't upset you, or answer the call for extra protein with other foods.

calcium

Your tiny offspring is growing bones and teeth and will pinch the very calcium out of your bones if you don't step up your intake. A calcium deficiency might mean you're more likely to get osteoporosis later in life. Many naturopaths say that calcium deficiency is one known cause of cramps, while many medical doctors say this is a fallacy and there's no scientific proof. If calcium helps your cramps, take it.

You'll probably need to have at least 1,600 milligrams of calcium a day during pregnancy (3 or 4 glasses of low-fat milk or servings of yogurt or cheese). This is about a third more than your non-pregnant requirement. Teenagers who are still growing themselves will need an especially high calcium allowance during pregnancy. Check with your dietician or doctor. Vitamin D is needed for efficient absorption of calcium, so a little bit of sunlight a day will help. You don't need a vitamin D supplement. Too much of this vitamin can be bad for you when pregnant.

Some examples of calcium-rich foods are dairy foods (milk, yogurt, and parmesan cheese in particular), spinach or other leafy green vegetables, broccoli, tofu, and fish. Some people want to get all their calcium needs from dairy products, not least because about 1 pound of cooked spinach or 2 pounds of cooked broccoli yields the same amount as a glass of milk. (This doesn't mean you can just drink gallons of milk and never eat your greens!) But if you want or need to avoid dairy products, your other calcium-packed options include sardines, canned salmon with the little bones in it, and tahini made from unhulled sesame seeds.

It's a good idea to maintain a calcium supplement (which ideally contains magnesium and zinc as well) while breast-feeding is making demands on your body's calcium supplies.

magnesium

You need magnesium or you don't get the full effect of the calcium and protein you take in. It's also used in therapeutic doses to combat preeclampsia—pregnancy-related high blood pressure (we'll get to that later in the book). Some good sources of magnesium are whole-wheat flour, muesli, wheat germ, beet leaves, chard, spinach, and raw parsley.

It's important to have magnesium included in a calcium supplement because of its crucial role in helping to retain calcium in bones and because normal diets are often deficient in magnesium.

zinc

Zinc needs to be increased during pregnancy and lactation (breastfeeding). Zinc is needed for enzyme production, for brain and nerve formation, and to help build an immune system in the fetus. Proper zinc levels have been linked to safer birth weights and less-premature babies. This mineral is often really low in pregnant women's diets. It's found in wheat bran, wheat germ, dried ginger, Brazil nuts, hazelnuts, peanuts (with lesser levels in other nuts), dried peas, and other legumes, red meat, chicken, fish, whole grains, and cheeses, especially Parmesan.

⚭ A zinc supplement is even more important if you're taking an iron supplement because iron may interfere with the body's absorption of zinc. Vegetarians and vegans especially may need a zinc supplement. A zinc supplement during breastfeeding is also often recommended.

folate (folic acid)

This B-group vitamin is now universally acknowledged as a supplement every woman should take for three months before pregnancy and for three months after conception. It has been proven dramatically effective in reducing neural tube defects by up to 70 percent—the main one is spina bifida—which affect 1 in 600 pregnancies. Although folate is naturally available in green leafy and yellow vegetables and whole-grain cereal, up to half of it can be lost in cooking or storage.

⊘ Just to cover yourself, it's best to take a supplement or prenatal vitamin rather than try to make up the folate requirement in food every day. A daily dose of at least 800 micrograms (μg)—not 800 milligrams (mg), the more common measurement of many supplements—is the recommended daily dose. Higher doses of folic acid are recommended if you've already had a pregnancy with a neural tube problem. When you buy the supplement, make sure you get at least 800 micrograms. If you're taking a multivitamin or mineral supplement that contains folate, check that there's at least 800 micrograms of it per daily dose: there usually isn't.

other B-group vitamins

Vegetarians and vegans will need to take vitamin B_{12} supplements or drink plenty of soy milk fortified with B_{12}. B_{12} only occurs naturally in animal products and is crucial in developing the baby's nervous system, brain, and red blood cells.

◊ A supplement containing B-group vitamins can be good for keeping up energy levels during pregnancy.

iron

Your iron requirement increases during the pregnancy: up to 20 percent of women become iron deficient during pregnancy. Extra blood volume—yours and the baby's—means more iron is needed to make more hemoglobin. The placenta gives first priority to the baby's iron requirements, taking it from your blood, and you risk anemia if you don't make up for it. You're considered to be at higher risk from iron deficiency if you're having a multiple pregnancy, you've had children quickly one after another, you've been vomiting a lot during pregnancy, or you're a vegetarian or vegan.

You need 22–36 milligrams per day during the last six months of pregnancy compared to a non-pregnant requirement of 12–16 milligrams. Iron absorption is helped by vitamin C and hindered by tea, coffee, and antacid medicines. You need to double or triple your usual amount of iron during the last 6 months of pregnancy. You should be getting 22–36 milligrams a day. Good sources of iron are lean beef, wheat bran, parsley, dried peaches, figs and apricots, spinach, sardines, and lentils.

⊘ Iron supplements are sometimes recommended from about the thirteenth week of pregnancy to keep up that daily requirement of 22–36 milligrams after the first trimester. Vegetarians who are not careful about their diet, and vegans, will need an iron supplement. Vegetarians will also find it very helpful when they don't feel like eating a mountain of spinach. Supplements may cause constipation, or sometimes diarrhea, and this should be discussed with your dietician, naturopath, midwife, or obstetrician, who can suggest an alternative form.

fats

You gotta have 'em for proper fetal development, but steer clear of saturated fats. Use monounsaturated vegetable oils, such as extra virgin olive oil, for cooking and salad dressings. You also need fatty acids, found in linseeds or linseed oil, pumpkin seeds, walnuts, pecans, and oily fish, and linoleic acid, found in seeds, seed and vegetable oils, nuts, and dark green vegetables. Avoid high-fat cooking methods such as frying and roasting in fat: better to grill, steam, and stir-fry.

sugar and salt

Going for nine months without any sugar is, of course, deeply weird. But do try to avoid refined sugars where possible, for all the usual reasons. (You probably already know that eating a block of chocolate the size of your head is not considered healthy.)

A completely salt-free diet isn't recommended, but there's enough natural salt in food without shaking on extra.

fluids

Get onto them! You'll have more blood pumping around and the amniotic fluid surrounding the developing baby is constantly being replaced. (Not to mention all that sweating and crying that can go on.) Drinking at least 2 quarts of water a day will help you avoid constipation and urinary tract infection. Steer clear of diuretics such as caffeine and alcohol. Diuretic drugs are unsafe during pregnancy, even if you have fluid retention: plain dandelion-leaf tea is okay (this is not the same as dandelion-root coffee substitute—dandelion-leaf tea looks more like a bag of bad marijuana or lawn clippings).

more info on eating and supplements

Try not to get obsessed about restrictive diets and panic about milligrams of this or that or weekly weight targets. Eat a varied diet with lots of protein, veggies, and fruit and for pete's sake don't start weighing anything!

Women's Trouble: Natural and Medical Solutions by Ruth Trickey and Kaz Cooke, Allen and Unwin, Sydney, 1998.

What a woman needs and why (apart from a masseur and chocolate ice cream). Covers all sorts of things that can go wrong with the girlie bits from ovarian cysts and period pain to PMS, endometriosis, and major surgery. Explores the herbal and medical options for each problem. Contains sensible guidelines on eating for health.

The nutritionists at your hospital, women's health center, or community health clinic will be able to help you. See Hospitals and Women's Information Services in Help.

PREGNANCY BOOKS

 A lot of books are handed to you when you're pregnant. Don't take them. When a friend recommends a book, buy the latest edition of it yourself. Some pregnancy books with out-of-date, even dangerous medical and safety info are passed around. And don't lend yours when you've finished with it. Here's a brief critical look at the main ones in circulation.

What to Expect When You're Expecting by Arlene Eisenberg, Heidi E. Murkoff, and Sandee E. Hathaway, Workman, New York, 2002.

Despite the stupid drawing on the front—which shows a woman in a rocking chair who looks like she's recovering from a lobotomy—this hefty paperback is a great pick-up-and-put-down, look-it-up-when-you-need-to pregnancy guide that includes things that can go wrong. If you've thought about it, developed it, or are worried about it, it's probably in this book somewhere.

Active Birth: The New Approach to Giving Birth Naturally by Janet Balaskas, Harvard Common Press, Boston, 1992.

Janet Balaskas is a long-time activist for the concept of active birth, in which the mother is in control of the labor situation, is able to move about, gives birth in an upright position (such as squatting or kneeling), and prepares for this during pregnancy with yoga and other natural methods. There is a manifesto about why this is so much better for mother's bodies and minds. (In the old days hospitals forced women to give birth on their backs with their legs in the air, working against gravity.) The book is full of yoga exercises demonstrated by women in horizontal-striped outfits, who look like very calm giant bees. There are lots of diagrams and photographs and explanations of active childbirth, and sections on home and hospital births, and post-natal issues and exercises. (Note: Make sure your obstetrician agrees with the principles of active birth if you are anticipating using this method. The book does not cover any medical intervention that may be really needed in the end, such as a cesarean. Not being able to have an active birth has nothing to do with you preparing wrongly. It's just the luck of the draw.)

New Natural Pregnancy: Practical Wellbeing from Conception to Birth by Janet Balaskas and Gayle Petersen, Interlink Pub Group, 1999.
Concentrating on the mother, a holistic look at pregnancy with sections on emotions, nutrition, yoga and exercise, massage, natural therapies, and holistic healing. Lots of illustrations of exercises, massage techniques, and natural remedies for common pregnancy complaints.

Conception, Pregnancy and Birth by Dr. Miriam Stoppard, DK Publishing, New York, 2000.
A large-format book with the best in-uterus photos, although I didn't think much of the text. It has an emphasis on body and beauty concerns as well as the usual pregnancy and birth stuff. Her previous pregnancy book has drawings that make the pregnant woman look like a demented robot having a bad-hair day.

Your Pregnancy Questions and Answers by Glade B. Curtis, consulting editor D. F. Hawkins, Perseus Publishing, Cambridge, MA, 2001.
Written by a couple of gynecologists, one English, one American. Hundreds of questions answered, but in a very brief way. Covers pregnancy, single moms, problems, nutrition, tests, childbirth, and feeding. A good one if you're anxious.

Pregnancy, Birth, and the Early Months: The Thinking Women's Guide by Richard Feinbloom, Perseus Publishing, Boston, 2000.
An experienced pediatrician, Feinbloom has written a sensible book on pregnancy with a detailed section on labor, pain relief, and things that can go wrong.

Preparing for Birth with Yoga by Janet Balaskas, Element Books, London, England, 1997.
All the women in the photos look very calm and supple. I say we kill them now.

your record

List the strategies you took to try to get pregnant, such as identifying ovulation. (If you *weren't* trying, why not record your method of contraception for posterity!) How long did you try for?

what's going on

Fertilization! Inside you your single-cell egg is tootling slowly down the fallopian tube when it is rather suddenly accosted by an insistent sperm, which wriggles inside it. The cell splits in two, then those two new cells split in two, and so on, within a surrounding jellylike coat. This fertilized egg, or embryo, takes about four days to languidly drift down the tube and into the uterus. A couple of days after arriving it finally sheds its jellylike coating and decides where to park itself, usually in the top, front part of the uterus. By now it's made up of about 200 cells. There's an innie bit that is the embryo, and an outie bit that will become the placenta (which will sustain the developing baby) and the amniotic sac (which contains the nice, warm amniotic-fluid "bath" the growing baby will float around in).

The embryo sends out roots to anchor it in the endometrium surface and draw in goodies from your bloodstream. It's this system that develops into the placenta.

DiARY We're getting ready to move house. I want
everything in its place. Tidy, tidy, tidy. I've been
collecting boxes and putting things in them and
pretending this means I'm an organized person
with a streamlined life. Actually it just means that I'm a
disorganized person in possession of a number of boxes.

Matt bought a small minivan to transport his palm trees,
ficuses, and, for really tasteful landscaping jobs, small statues of
peeing cherubs. This vehicular purchase, along with moving to a
larger house, has led to much unseemly speculation. Combine real
estate move, larger car, and a hint of an enigmatic smile, which
one cultivates to cover a whirling sense of nothing-to-speak-of
going on in the brainish region, and there is an immediate bun-in-
the-oven calculation on the part of bystanders.

Some people, almost always the ones who have their own kids
and often plenty of them, bang on about it constantly. "Are you
pregnant yet?" "When are you going to start a family?" as if a
baby's just something you send off for with a stamped, self-
addressed envelope.

Luckily we don't have the sort of parents who pressure us,
given that Mom died before I could remember her and nobody
knows who my dad was, and Matt's parents are usually off
studying lichen in the most bio-eccentric mountains of Venezuela
rather than demanding that we have some grandchildren to keep
them amused. I am constantly amazed by the parents of friends
who think it's their perfect right to insist that their offspring hurry
up and "give them grandchildren."

I'm sure Aunt Peg, who raised me with the help of Uncle Stan
before he ran off with that belly dancer from Niagara Falls . . .
what was her name? Mandii the Magnificent was on the posters,
but I'm pretty sure she made the last bit up . . . anyway, I'm sure
Aunt Peg would be rapt, but at least she isn't leaning on me. Uncle
Stan, who has become a born-again retired-hippie, would no
doubt go all new-age on me. And he ought to know by now I'm
not the Earth Mother type.

Just for fun, Matt and I have been playing parents with a
Tamagotchi baby we found at a garage sale—it's one of those tiny

Japanese digital games that look like key rings. We turned the game on, called our electronic-screen baby Fred and pressed Start. There was a button to be pressed when Fred produced what the instructions called "dung" and buttons to press to see Fred's weight and age; to play paper, scissors, rock with him; to give him rice or a bottle; and to "discipline" him. (Unfortunately there seemed to be no Child Protective Services button.)

Every night Matt bounds in from a day of demanding clients saying things like, "What about a daiquiri fountain on the east lawn?" and "I've never liked agapanthus" and "Can't we just concrete that bit?" and "No, I've changed my mind," and he asks breathlessly and tenderly, "How's Fred?"

And each time, flushed with the bloom of mothering a newborn, baby-purple extruded-plastic capsule with digital liquid-crystal output screen thingie, I report, "Haven't seen him all day. Busy," "Try the silverware drawer," or "I left him in a café." Or more often, the simply poignant diagnosis, "Well . . . Fred's dead." Damn depressing game, if you ask me.

No, it has to be said: motherhood is the hardest and most honorable job in the world. Oh, well. With my medical history it might take years to get pregnant. If at all. Probably just as well. Let's face it, I'm not likely to get a reference from Fred.

I suppose if I'm going to stay off the Pill, I had better find a friend with a baby and spend a day or so with them. I was off wearing miniskirts in exotic locales when Amanda's babies were small, and not that interested really. Now that I am, I realize most of my friends are lesbians or career women who are only just starting to wonder how they might manage it. The only one who's already launched her kayak into the creek is Marg, and she's only four months pregnant. I guess I can practice on her baby when it arrives. I had better find an instructional video called something like *A New Baby: Which End Up?*

We just don't live anymore in a tribal society surrounded by a million kids of various ages and great numbers of extended families. My second cousin Hank has six of the monsters, but they live on the other side of the globe so there's not much practicing to be had there. There should be some kind of library service.

info

sense of smell

Your sense of smell may be far more acute than usual during pregnancy, especially in the first three months. You may even notice it before you know you're pregnant. Perfumes or food smells that previously seemed downright scrumptious may now send you heaving to the bathroom. What's really annoying is that none of the experts seem to be able to say why. Maybe the nausea is a defense mechanism so you're more likely to identify "off" foods that could harm you or your baby. Maybe it's to compensate for the last two-thirds of a pregnancy often being accompanied by a blocked nose (due to a general increase in bodily secretions you don't want to have to think about yet). Or maybe it's just a meaningless side effect of one of the pregnancy hormones.

aromatherapy

Aromatherapy, the therapeutic use of essential oils, can make you feel nurtured and relaxed during pregnancy, but some essential oils can harm your unborn baby or bring on labor or even a miscarriage, especially if applied directly to the skin during a bath or massage.

Qualified aromatherapists advise against any aromatherapy being applied directly to the skin in this way during pregnancy, especially during the first trimester, without advice from an aromatherapist specializing in pregnancy. Some oils are not even recommended for burning to scent a room when you're pregnant.

Unfortunately some masseurs who use essential oils without being qualified aromatherapists are simply unaware of any risks and will tell you anything they use is quite safe at whatever concentration they feel like squirting on you. And even the oils considered "safe" for massage or in the bath should be used at half strength during pregnancy.

It can be confusing for a layperson to decide what is safe. For example, despite the fact that spearmint used directly on the skin appears in the "banned during pregnancy" list given below, some pregnancy magazines recommend it to relieve nausea when used as an infusion to breathe in or to scent a room.

Oils generally considered safe for use during pregnancy include lavender, grapefruit, orange, lemon, tangerine, mandarin, neroli, sandalwood, ylang-ylang, geranium (after the fifth month), bergamot, ginger, and tea tree.

Oils that can induce miscarriage (abortifacients) or bring on a period (emmenagogues) must be avoided during pregnancy. They include, but may not be exclusively confined to, yarrow, aniseed, tarragon, caraway, atlas cedarwood, camphor, hyssop, pennyroyal, spearmint, parsley and parsley seed, rosemary, nutmeg, Roman chamomile, German chamomile, myrrh, juniper, lovage, peppermint, basil, Spanish marjoram, clary sage, sage, bay, vetiver, pine, thyme, jasmine, wintergreen, and angelica.

Remember that you may be supersensitive to smell, but your nose can also be blocked up during pregnancy and therefore *less* sensitive to smell. So always follow the recipes given by a qualified aromatherapist rather than your schnozz. And obviously, for your own comfort, don't use anything that makes you feel queasy.

Here are some safe aromatherapy ideas.

⊚ Aches and pains—throw a couple of drops of lavender oil in the bath.

⊚ Fatigue—in a burner to send the smell wafting through the room, 2 drops of lavender oil, put 1 drop of mandarin oil, and 1 drop of ylang-ylang oil; or 1 drop of lavender oil, 1 drop of mandarin oil, and 2 drops of ylang-ylang oil.

⑥ Nausea—in a burner, put 1–2 drops of lemon oil or lemongrass oil; or drink some ginger tea (see Nausea in Week 4) and breathe in the aroma as you go.

⑥ Insomnia—put 3 drops of lavender, mandarin, or ylang-ylang oil, or a mixture of the three, in the bath; or scent your bedroom with 2–3 drops of lavender or ylang-ylang oil, or a mixture of the two.

⑥ Stuffy nose—make an inhalation by adding 2 drops of eucalyptus or tea-tree oil to a bowl of hot water, then stick a towel over your head and breathe in the vapor for a couple of minutes. (You can't use many "cold remedy" drugs during pregnancy so this is a good one to remember.)

⑥ Bad circulation—in a burner, put 2 drops of grapefruit oil, eucalyptus oil, or frankincense.

Aromatherapy won't actually help with pain relief during labor and naked flames are banned in hospitals, by the way.

herbal teas

Many herbs can bring on a period or cause miscarriage or birth defects. Always check with a trained herbalist. (No more than three cups of any kind of herbal tea should be consumed every day as a habit.)

Herbal teas that are generally considered safe during pregnancy include peppermint, fresh ginger, lemon balm, chamomile, and dandelion leaf (which is a safe diuretic) but not dandelion root. Herbal teas should not be confused with essential oils: an oil extracted from a plant contains very large quantities of components that could be dangerous, whereas a tea made from the plant might not.

medicine and natural therapies

Remember, don't take medications, herbs, or vitamins without consulting a properly trained doctor or herbalist. Just because your friend took something during her pregnancy that she swears by doesn't mean it's safe for you or your baby. Some preparations can be taken at different times during the pregnancy; others are dangerous at certain times, or at any stage. Some preparations are safe *except* during pregnancy. Don't assume because something is "natural" it is safe. And always tell your doctor and naturopath what the other one has prescribed.

Beware of dippy "natural therapy" or diet advice. Most diets that involve restriction of certain food types are not suitable for pregnancy, and fasting is compleeeeetely out of the question as it could damage the developing baby or even cause miscarriage. (See Eating and Supplements in Week 2 for the lowdown on eating during pregnancy.)

WEEK 4

what's going on

Your period is due. Maybe you've started going pee, pee, pee all the way home. Perhaps you've gone off the smell of alcohol and cigarettes, and foods that you usually like. Now or in the next few weeks, you might start feeling slightly queasy, which in bad cases results in vomiting. (According to one pregnancy book photo, this is when you will wear a hideous smock and a headband and stare out the window holding a cup and saucer like a demented fool.)

The tiny embryo burrows into the wall of the uterus until it's completely embedded, and it keeps getting bigger every day. The ovaries are pumping out the hormone progesterone to make the endometrium tough. The sex of your baby, the color of its hair and eyes, how tall it can grow and whether it has natural soccer talent—all these factors have been genetically programmed from the start and can't be altered. By the end of this week the embryo's about a fifth of a millimeter—still too little to see without using magnifying instruments.

glamour
glamour
glamour

DIARY Went for a drink with my old pal Juan, whose wife has been at home with the kids for four years and is now dashing her head against a plywood wall trying to get into the workforce again—the restaurant industry wants her to work split shifts for approximately 75 cents a day. He says apart from this whole work problem, and vomit and poop, motherhood is INCREDIBLY GLAMOUROUS.

I meet with the boss about becoming head designer of Real Women Wear and agree to a schedule of sacred weekly meetings with the new buyers. I sign the contract for my first line. Off to Betsy's party with the girls and smoke about seven cigarettes— and have two glasses of killer punch. For some reason I don't want to get drunk. Have a bit of a half-hearted dance. I'm feeling kind of tired and out of sorts. Not quite nauseous but squirgly in the tummy.

For some reason I've started being absolutely vile to Matt. I don't know why. I'm quite aware I'm doing it but I can't stop myself: I am the Bitch Queen of the Universe. He comes in the front door and I narrow my eyes looking for a fault. I swear if he came in the door with a bunch of mauve roses and tickets to the Bahamas I'd probably say, "Wipe those filthy boots!" for all the world as if I had suddenly developed a passion for clean floors. I'm really starting to worry. I think I'm turning into a drill sergeant.

Oh, how could I be so STUPID? It must be PMS. I've just forgotten what it's like after four years on the Pill.

info

nausea

Some people still call it morning sickness, but it isn't, so they shouldn't. It can get you at any time of the day, even all day. Not everybody gets it, but most pregnant women experience some form of nausea, usually in the first trimester, and half will throw up at least once. It can range from a slightly queasy feeling to full-on, head-in-a-bucket, serious vomiting. For some very unlucky women, it persists after week 14, even all through the pregnancy.

The cause has not been absolutely identified and may even vary from person to person. The culprits are thought to include any or all of the following: high levels of the hormone HCG; a fall in blood pressure resulting from progesterone-induced relaxation of muscles, which causes dilation of the blood vessels; less-efficient digestion due to less stomach acid in the gut; an increase in estrogen challenging the liver to break it down, so the liver works overtime; and altered senses, which means that some smells and tastes make you feel sick. (For more info see Pregnancy Hormones in Week 12.)

Here are some things that may help.

⑥ Eat small, frequent snacks to avoid an empty tummy or a low blood-sugar level—keep a handbag or briefcase pantry of crackers, nuts, and dried or fresh fruits and vegetables.

⑥ Have four or five smaller meals a day instead of three biggies (this can also be useful in the third trimester when your tummy is squished up).

⑥ Eat something bland *before* you get out of bed in the morning, such as dry toast or a cracker, or have a small amount of fruit juice.

⑥ Have a snack just before bedtime.

⑥ Avoid the fish market or perfume counter or anything else that makes you feel queasy; this can include fatty or fried foods, cigarette smoke, coffee, and alcohol.

⑥ Maintain your intake of protein (chicken soup is good) and complex carbohydrates (potato, rice, and pasta).

⑥ Avoid getting tired or stressed.

⑥ Try ginger tea—infuse 1–2 teaspoons of grated fresh ginger (or a piece of ginger, about the size of your little finger and chopped into four or five bits) in a small teapot of boiling water for 5 minutes; strain; add honey or a squeeze of lemon to taste, breathing in the steam as you go.

◎ Sniff a fresh lemon.

◎ If you've been vomiting, drink lots of water so you don't become dehydrated.

◎ Try vitamin B$_6$ (less than 500 milligrams per day), which may be recommended by naturopaths and doctors for severe sickness.

It's not common for vomiting to be so bad that it needs medical intervention, but if you are vomiting more than once a day for several days in a row, or any aspect of your vomiting is distressing, tell your doctor right away. The main risks are that you may dehydrate, especially if you can't keep down fluids, and that the baby may miss out on nutrients.

Nausea is often said to be a good sign—evidence that the hormones are pumping, indicating a strong, stable pregnancy. Some people claim that first-trimester nausea indicates a lower risk of miscarriage. (Others point out that nausea affects only half of all pregnant women, so it's hardly a prerequisite for a healthy pregnancy.) More severe nausea can be associated with a twin or multiple pregnancy because the hormone levels in the bloodstream are higher.

looking after your embryo and fetus

Teratogens are infections, substances, or environmental factors that can damage an embryo or fetus at certain stages of development—the biggest danger being in the first three months of pregnancy. (In usual tactless-doctor language, *teratogen* is derived from the ancient Greek *teras,* meaning monster.) The effect of teratogens can range from impaired growth or increased risk of a miscarriage to serious birth defects.

The impact on the developing baby depends on the teratogen—some are much more dangerous than others—and your level of exposure, as well as what stage of pregnancy you're at when exposed, individual susceptibility, and luck. (Even if you know somebody who drank vodka like a mad thing through their pregnancy and had a "normal baby," it doesn't mean the same will apply to you.)

It's believed that not much damage is likely to be done between conception and when the egg implants itself in the wall of the uterus 6 to 8 days later. The most dangerous time is from implantation to the tenth week after conception, when major organs and limbs are being formed. But some teratogens can affect major parts of the developing baby throughout the whole pregnancy, including the brain, eyes, and sex organs.

scary illnesses

Hyperthermia (overheating) Any illness that causes a high temperature (101°F or more) for an extended time, especially in the first 3 months of pregnancy, can cause damage to an embryo or fetus.

Toxoplasmosis This illness can be symptomless or feel like mild flu. It's caused by a parasite commonly found in raw or under-cooked meat (meat should be cooked to an internal temperature of at least 140°F), including poultry; unpasteurized goat's milk products; and the poop from cats and, more rarely, dogs. The infection can cause brain and eye damage in the fetus, and miscarriage. The greatest period of risk is the third trimester. Many people come into contact with the parasite at some point during their life and develop an immunity to it.

Avoid cats if possible. If you have a cat, have someone else in the household empty the litterbox, or use gloves if you do it. Wash your hands after touching a cat. Wear gloves when gardening. Before eating raw, garden-grown produce, wash it thoroughly with soap and hot water.

Listeriosis This relatively rare bacterial infection is transmitted through foods. Its symptoms include fever, headache, tiredness, aches, and pains. It may cause miscarriage or stillbirth. High-risk foods are "ready-to-eat" seafood, such as smoked fish and mussels (but canned fish should be safe); bagged salad mixes; deli meats; precooked meats and pâtés; milkshakes and soft-serve ice-cream; and unpasteurized milk or milk products, especially soft cheeses such as brie, blue cheese, and Camembert.

Rubella (German measles) Rubella can cause a high incidence of abnormalities in babies (congenital rubella syndrome includes blindness and deafness), particularly when mothers are exposed to it in the first trimester. Nevertheless, the disease is rare in the United States because most people have been vaccinated against it. Often you need a booster shot, so before trying to get pregnant it's a good idea to have your doctor order a blood test to check your immunity. If you need to be vaccinated, wait 3 months afterward before trying to conceive, so your system has time to destroy the live virus in the vaccine. Your obstetrician will order a rubella test for you if you're already pregnant to check your immunity status.

Syphilis This increasingly uncommon sexually transmitted disease (STD) can cross the placenta and cause premature birth, stillbirth, or long-term effects in children such as dental abnormalities. It can be detected in routine pregnancy tests and safely treated in early pregnancy. It can also infect the baby during the birth, and the baby can then be cured with drugs.

Chlamydia An STD that can be associated with ear infection and/or pneumonia of the baby. Chlamydia can easily be cured with antibiotics.

Gonorrhea Another STD, gonorrhea can also infect the baby during the birth, and the baby can then be cured with drugs.

Human immunodeficiency virus (HIV) Pregnant women with HIV will not automatically pass it on to their babies. Estimates of transmission range from 14 to 50 percent. Mothers with HIV must not breastfeed, as transmission rates are much higher. (This is why infant formula is once again being promoted by health workers in Africa.)

Genital herpes An active case can infect the baby during birth. If you have genital herpes, your obstetrician should closely monitor it in the latter part of the pregnancy. If you have an active case at the time of delivery, a cesarean section done within four hours of breaking your water will most likely protect your baby from possible infection. If you have a history of genital herpes, your doctor may prescribe an anti-viral medicine during the last four weeks of your pregnancy to decrease the chance of your having an infection at the time of labor.

Cytomegalovirus (CMV) The most common infectious cause of mental retardation and congenital deafness, cytomegalovirus is a virus that can be transmitted through young children. If you work in a daycare or hospital, be sure to wash your hands frequently.

Hepatitis C and B It is believed that very few pregnant women with hep C will have babies who are infected. There are only a few case studies so far, but it is thought that babies are more likely to get hep C if their mom was exposed to it in the third trimester. There is some suggestion that transmission is more likely if the mom has HIV as well. If you have any history of intraveneous drug use or blood transfusion, ask your doctor to test you for the hep C and hep B antibodies.

Other diseases and conditions There are many diseases and conditions that can affect your embryo or fetus. Some of these have "silent" symptoms so you may not be aware of any risk or problem.

Tell your doctor about any high fever, rash, sweating, or fluid retention during your pregnancy or any other symptom that worries you.

what goes in: dangerous substances

No prescription or over-the-counter drug, herbal or natural remedy, or vitamin or mineral supplement should be taken during pregnancy without consulting a doctor who knows you're pregnant. No recreational or street drugs are safe to use during pregnancy. (But it can be even more dangerous to try to quit an addiction to heroin, for example, during the pregnancy—see below.) It's a good idea to get clean before you conceive, and you can get help to stay that way. Many people think that knowing they're having a baby will get them to quit drugs or alcohol, but that's rarely enough. Everyone needs help to quit an addiction, and help is available. Make sure you tell your doctor about any drugs you've used during pregnancy.

Vitamin A Any supplement or acne or skin treatment containing vitamin A should be stopped while you're pregnant, and avoid liver and liver products such as pâté.

Caffeine An intake of 3 or more cups of tea or coffee a day is associated with low birth weight and may double, some say triple, the risk of miscarriage in the first trimester. The same is true of cola drinks.

Alcohol Nobody knows the safe amount you can have, so complete avoidance is usually recommended. It is said that excessive daily drinking or binge drinking can cause fetal alcohol syndrome: mental retardation, slow growth, and a variety of physical abnormalities and behavioral problems. Excessive drinking during pregnancy has been variously defined, from more than two drinks a day to any alcohol at all.

Cigarettes Cigarette smoking and using other tobacco products stunts the growth of the fetus. This has been an "excuse" for women who keep smoking while pregnant ("It'll be an easier birth if it's a small baby"). But smoking also inhibits the growth of the placenta and is believed to be linked to miscarriage, stillbirth, sudden infant death syndrome (SIDS), childhood asthma, and other respiratory traumas for babies and children. Second-hand smoke should also be avoided. If your partner smokes, suggest that this would be the best time to quit. Or at least, do not allow your partner to smoke inside of your home or car. There are many programs and even some drugs which are safe to use during pregnancy to help pregnant women stop smoking.

Marijuana and hashish   Their use is linked to premature birth and low birth weight. There is no known "safe" amount.

LSD and other hallucinogens   LSD use carries the risk of miscarriage and chromosomal damage. There is little research on other hallucinogens but it's safest to assume any amount is dangerous.

Ecstasy   There isn't much detailed research yet on "newer" recreational drugs—although ecstasy has been associated with increased risk of placental bleeding—but we know they're definitely not a good idea to use when you're pregnant.

Amphetamines (speed)   Speed is associated with premature babies and possibly baby heart problems.

Heroin and methadone   These drugs can cause prematurity, low birth weight, mental problems, and stillbirth. Babies share their mother's addiction and so suffer withdrawal symptoms when they are born, although this can be managed by medical staff usually over a matter of weeks. Taking prescribed methadone is preferable to using heroin in pregnancy because it provides a regulated dose to the fetus. The baby must be weaned from its methadone addiction after birth. Coming off heroin suddenly while pregnant is a cause of miscarriage: don't stop abruptly without talking to your doctor.

Cocaine   Even a single, one-time dose can damage a fetus.

environmental hazards

If your job or workplace is unsafe during pregnancy, you have the legal right to be given duties that don't expose you to the hazards. Avoid any of the following.

Radiation X-rays can cause malformations in a fetus. Tell any doctor or dentist who wants to X-ray you that you're pregnant. If you had one before you knew you were pregnant, ask your obstetrician about the risk to the fetus. It's usually not bad news. Low-level radiation emitted by computer visual display units has not been proven to have an effect on a pregnancy or a developing baby.

Getting too hot As with overheating caused by illness, your body temperature should not be above 101°F for an extended time. Avoid hot tubs and steam rooms.

Poisons and pesticides There are heaps of potentially harmful substances at home and in the workplace. Read labels and avoid using toxins. Definitely avoid "fumy" cleaning products, including oven cleaners and dry-cleaning solvents, most paints, lacquers, thinners, paint strippers, pesticides, herbicides, gasoline, glue, many manufacturing chemicals and waste products. Beware of lead in the air in heavy traffic areas and nearby soil, in old house paint and in some water, particularly in houses with old lead pipes or lead-soldered pipes. Lead can also leach into food or drink from very old or handmade china or earthenware pottery.

People in high-risk jobs include health-care workers, farmers, gardeners, factory workers, printing or photographic processing workers, artists, chemists, hairdressers, nail artists, dry cleaners, cleaners, and people who work with gasoline. Exposure to air pollution—such as carbon monoxide from car exhaust and smoke from cigarettes—may be a problem if your job involves driving in heavy traffic for much of the day, directing traffic, working at a bus station, or working at a venue filled with cigarette smoke, such as a bar.

Unfortunately, the list of potentially harmful substances you might come into contact with is extensive. Fortunately, most babies turn out fine anyway. To find out whether substances or practices specific to your circumstances are harmful during pregnancy, make sure you check with your doctor, the Occupational Safety and Health Administration (OSHA), or union. You mustn't rely on your employer as the only source of information about what's in your workplace and what the risks are to you.

TELL YOUR DOCTOR RIGHT AWAY ABOUT ANY:

- bleeding from the vagina.
- vomiting, if you can't keep down fluids.
- abdominal pain.
- repeated fainting spells.
- high temperature.
- major fluid retention.
- worries, including depression.
- instruction or information they gave you that you don't fully understand.
- really funny baby jokes you've heard.

1

2

3

4

5

6

7

8

what's going on Your period hasn't turned

up. You might feel premenstrual, with slightly swollen breasts,

as well as peeing more often and feeling queasy.

The embryo is still very tiny but starting to form into a

tube shape and growing very quickly. The head and tail ends

become obvious. The heart and blood vessels are only just

starting to form so the embryo doesn't have its independent

circulation yet. At this stage the placenta consists of lots of

"tentacles" called chorionic villi. Eventually they will grow into the

big, temporary organ that runs the exchange between you

and your developing baby, which sends in nutrients and oxygen

and takes out waste products and carbon dioxide, using the

vein and two arteries in the umbilical cord that connects

it to the baby. You'll find that pregnancy books disagree on

the size of the developing baby, partly because some

measure from head to butt, and some from

head to feet.

Diary We move and my thirty-third birthday party on Sunday is conducted amid towers of cardboard boxes and chests full of stuff we didn't even open at the last house. My advice to anyone under 27 is don't blink or you'll be 33 before you know what happened. Kind of like Rumpelstiltskin. (Only your beard isn't usually *quite* that bad.)

People at the party keep asking, "Maddie, do you want another drink?" and I keep saying no. Just like that. No, meaning no, I don't want a drink, which means people keep looking at me strangely. Or I say yes and then leave the drink somewhere under a tree.

And it is really pricey champagne too, being my birthday and everybody being nice about it. And normally, although I don't smoke—except other people's (oh, all right, and those times when I buy a pack for a party . . . yes, and those other times when . . . oh, shut up)—I will have the odd puff at a social extravaganza, even one involving moving boxes. But this time I just don't feel like it. Begin to feel quite snappy, and restless. All sort of "It's my party and I'll pout if I want to."

Then I get scared. I start to think: 33. Thirty-three and I don't want to party any more. It's over. It's been over since Matt bought that minivan. What was I thinking—that I could live in a house with a perfectly nice man who owns a minivan and has a steady job and earns his own money and doesn't expect me to pay for everything and isn't some kind of frustrated troll of a tortured artiste?

What happened to my life? When did I get sensible? How can I escape? Maybe I should run through the streets stark naked spitting at streetlights. Or I could just go to bed. I'm exhausted and my stomach has been squirgly again. Must be coming down with something. Need a good night's rest, probably. Nightie-night everyone. Please. Don't stop drinking on my account. I'll just zzzzzzzz.

4 A.M. Hang on a minute.

9:10 A.M. Pop down to the drugstore. Need some dental floss, some cotton balls, some orange nail polish, naturally, and, oh, what the hell, I'll take that $17 home pregnancy test kit on a whim.

Pregnancy tests from the drugstore have obviously changed since I was last a careless idiot. You used to have to pee into some sort of container (jelly jar, bucket, beer stein with "Lubbock Rodeo" written on the side of it, that kind of thing), and then dip a white plastic magic wand, which was a bit like a ballpoint pen, into it. The most useful instruction was always "Use the midstream urine for the test." What that meant was that you did some pee, then you stopped, if you had pelvic-floor muscles like a steel trap, and neatly did a mighty bull's-eye midstream pee into the jar, then stopped (steel trap again), removed the jar, and finished the pee.

What always happened was more like sticking a thimble under a waterfall and then snatching it out again and finding that, although you had pee on your hand, the outside of the jar, your hair, the cuffs of your pants, and some articles in another room entirely, you'd managed to miss the jar.

Now you're supposed to hold the magic wand in one hand and—I'm sorry, but basically you just piss on it for a minute or so. This seems such an incredibly male thing to do. I almost feel like trying to write my name in the snow with my own urine. But there is no snow. Only a thin, blue line showing in the window, which the instructions say means you're pregnant. And I'm not talking a baby blue, a wimpy sort of a "We think it's within the realm of possibility that you might conceivably have conceived." No, it is almost a luminous, pulsating navy blue indicating "YOU, madam, have a BUN IN THE OVEN for sure!"

I always thought I might cry a tiny tear of feminine yet sensible joy. Instead, I stare at the wall thinking, "Oh . . . Woo."

Call Matt and tell him to come straight home from water polo practice, there is something I have to tell him.

"Ooohhhh," he says, "Woo," sounding like he knows what it might be.

I tell him at the front door. He looks pretty shocked. We just start laughing, with tears in our eyes, and then we can't stop laughing. It just seems so ridiculously UNLIKELY. Matt says he is happy and then talks about the finer points of water polo really fast for about 25 minutes. I think he's in shock.

"You told me it would probably take two years to get pregnant," he says later, quietly.

"Ooops. Woo," I concur.

Matt commences to grin for two days straight, the grin punctuated by an expression of profound bewilderment. I begin to refer to him as the bewilderbeest. Luckily he's an optimist whose most remarkable traits include a "she'll be just fine" attitude to almost anything. If you told Matt there was a hurricane coming, he'd be dead interested from a meteorological point of view.

info

pregnancy tests

Home pregnancy test kits bought at the drugstore work the same way as a test a doctor would do on a sample of your pee. The kits test for the presence of HCG (human chorionic gonadotrophin hormone). The first pee of the day will have the greatest concentration of HCG.

You can do the test as early as 14 days after conception, about when your period would be due. Results of these tests are almost always accurate, especially if they're positive. A false negative result can happen if the levels of HCG being produced by a pregnant body are low. So if your period doesn't start, and you still suspect you are pregnant, you can wait a few days and do the test again, or go to the doctor for a blood test, which can measure HCG levels as early as 1 week after conception.

After a positive home test, or other signs of early pregnancy such as a missed period, tender breasts, nausea, frenzied peeing, a funny metallic taste in your mouth, tiredness, or moodiness, you should go to your health care provider for a physical examination. The doctor should be able to confirm the pregnancy and see further signs such as an enlarged uterus and the changed texture and color of the cervix (the small opening, and surrounding tissue, between the uterus and the vagina).

Depending on your medical history your health care provider might refer you to an obstetrician, a midwife, or a perinatologist who specializes in high-risk pregnancies.

ectopic pregnancy scan

When the pregnancy is confirmed, an early ultrasound scan might be recommended, if the doctor suspects you have an ectopic pregnancy, which happens when the embryo implants itself outside the uterus, usually in a tube. Sadly, an ectopic pregnancy can't be saved and turned into a viable pregnancy. Unless the body naturally aborts the embryo very early, it is a very serious medical problem and must be resolved by surgery as soon as it is diagnosed.

Risk factors include a previous ectopic pregnancy; pelvic inflammatory disease; damage to or scarring of the fallopian tubes caused by infection or surgery; endometriosis; an intra-uterine device (IUD) in place when you conceived; and your mom, when she was pregnant with you, having taken a morning-sickness drug called DES (diethylstilboestrol), which causes malformation of the reproductive organs in some babies.

Symptoms of ectopic pregnancy, which usually occur at about 6 weeks, may include abdominal pain, either on one side of the abdomen or more generalized, that can come and go; spotting or bleeding; dizziness, faintness, paleness, and sweating; nausea and vomiting; sometimes shoulder pain; and sometimes a feeling of pressure in the butt.

Tell your doctor or obstetrician immediately about these symptoms. Early treatment improves your chances of saving the tube and maintaining fertility. If a fallopian tube bursts, the pain is terrible: go straight to hospital because you'll need emergency surgery. Remember, it's definitely possible to have an ectopic pregnancy even if you think you can't conceive because you're on the Pill or Minipill.

routine tests

At your first obstetric appointment—and usually the longest— they'll compile a comprehensive medical history, noting details of your previous illnesses and surgeries; your allergies; prescription medications or alternative treatments you're taking; gynecological and obstetric history, including the pattern of your menstrual cycle; any STDs, past pregnancies, miscarriages, or pregnancy terminations (abortions); family history of twins or genetic disorders; your lifestyle, particularly your diet, smoking, drinking, drugs, work, and fitness habits; current or past depression; current or past experience with domestic violence; your family's medical history, and perhaps even your mom's obstetric history. Even so, most doctors nowadays understand that your mother's obstetric history is neither here nor there. How long your mother was in labor, whether she had nausea, what size you were as a baby, all that stuff is more than likely to be completely irrelevant to your own experience of pregnancy.

The routine tests probably include:

⊚ an internal examination to confirm the pregnancy and some chatting to estimate the delivery due date.

⊚ weighing you.

⊚ a Pap smear (in which some tiny cells are collected from your cervix).

⊚ basically a bit of an all-around physical—an examination of your heartbeat, lungs, blood pressure, pelvis, and abdomen.

⑥ examination of breasts and nipples.

⑥ a urine test to rule out a urinary tract infection.

⑥ a blood test to establish your blood type; possible anemia, and immunity to rubella and hepatitis; and history of syphilis. HIV testing is now also offered to all women.

Usually you visit the obstetrician monthly until late in the pregnancy, after which visits become bimonthly, and then weekly close to delivery.

As a routine at each visit your blood pressure will be checked and your tummy examined to measure the growth of the uterus, and you'll probably be weighed and have a urine test. After about 12 weeks you'll be able to hear the heartbeat when the obstetrician puts a listening device (often a Doppler ultrasound) on your tummy.

It's easy to forget something you've been meaning to ask the obstetrician—list your questions somewhere in your diary as they occur to you, and jot down the answers while you're there, too, because sometimes your head's in a whirl with all the new info and you can't remember them afterward.

WEEK

would you like a cup of tea?

what's going on

You can consider visiting your doctor and dating the

pregnancy—meaning: work out when you conceived.

(This is different from dating during pregnancy, an

activity that is often curtailed, especially in the last

few months.) If you haven't already, you may start to

feel grumpy or nauseated.

The embryo is growing rapidly and beginning to look

tadpoley. The tadpole tail will eventually shrink and the remnants

become the baby's coccyx. In the center of the embryo is the

6

start of the digestive system, lungs, and bladder. This is surrounded by a layer that will develop into muscles, skeleton, heart, kidneys, and genitals, and this is wrapped up in what will become the skin, nervous system, ears, and eyes. Tiny bumps are appearing that will grow into arms. The immature heart starts to beat and pump blood around the embryo and into the chorionic villi (the pre-placenta) and can be clearly seen as a pulsation on an ultrasound screen. Really, the whole thing looks like some tiny thing that might come out if you sneezed.

yeah? You and whose army?

Average approximate embryo length this week from head to butt

in

1

2

3

4

5

6

7

8

DiARY Work is heating up. We sign to produce two new fashion lines for a couple of big department stores. The spicy earth colors of winter! The divine madness of spring! You know the sort of thing. Will we get it all done before the baby arrives? I can't even tell anyone I'm pregnant yet. The convention is to wait until after 13 weeks, when they reckon the biggest risk of miscarriage is over.

We tell some close friends of Matt's, quietly, at a wedding. They scream. I have to pretend there is a spider down my underpants to explain the commotion.

I now know why horoscopes are a dead loss. You'd think they could warn you: "This week you'll get put in the family way." No, mine just said: "Financial difficulties may arise on Tuesday. Your lucky color is caramel." Nobody's lucky color is caramel. It's not even a color—it's half a meal.

Beck says I need to get my doctor to refer me to an obstetrician right away because of my endometriosis, which can cause an ectopic pregnancy. I call an obstetrician who she thinks is excellent. She heard this guy had a pretty good attitude. What clinched it for her was seeing him on TV the year he was the doctor who had delivered the most babies born to heroin-addicted moms. A journalist made a disparaging comment about the mothers, and he gently cradled a baby in his arms and said something that displayed general decency and compassion. His name is quite nerdy—Herb—which is strangely reassuring also. Maybe I'm becoming conservative in my old age, but I just don't want an obstetrician called Sparky.

I explain my medical history to Dr. Herb's receptionist/nurse who is almost certainly called Lorraine. All the sensible women I meet I automatically think of as Lorraines. Lorraines never wear high heels and they always know everything about their specialty, whether it's knitting, delivering babies, running a doctor's office, or basketball strategy.

Before I get to meet Dr. Herb, I have to have an ultrasound to check that the pregnant bit of me is where it should be—in the uterus—instead of ectopic (stuck in a fallopian tube), which can be very dangerous. So I go across the street to discover that my first ultrasound appointment means sitting in the waiting room for approximately 738 HOURS filling in a DAMN FORM.

Who is your family doctor? Haven't got one.

Last period? Well, in my case about 4 years, but surely that's going to take too long to explain.

Number of previous pregnancies? One. Well, therein lies *another* story, but do they really want to hear about the anesthesiologist who wanted to get the abortion over with so he could get to the soccer game on time? Probably not. Nor, I feel sure, do they want to know about the ex-boyfriend who threw a check on the kitchen table in front of housemates and visitors, saying, "That's for my half of the abortion," and then refused to speak to me ever again. This pregnancy business sure flicks open the clasps on your emotional baggage.

I look at the posters on the wall of a fetus developing week by week. It was so long ago. I can't remember now whether I terminated at 6 weeks or 8 weeks. So many of us women having babies in our thirties had abortions when we were younger, vowing that we would only become mothers when we could be good at it. I'm glad I waited. I didn't even know who I really was then. But I really don't want to look at that poster.

Previous surgery: how many operations? Can't remember so compromise by writing "Loads." That should give 'em the general idea.

Husband's name? Haven't got one. Well, I have got a boyfriend. Must be worse for Marg when she fills out these kinds of forms. I mean, what is a single girl like her supposed to write? Missing in Action? NA (Not Available)? NOYB (None of Your Business)? Or just Albert Einstein?

I go into a small room and lie on a flat, hard, raised couch. The ultrasound operator, Dr. Donaldson, sits next to me at about hip level with a screen in front of him and a nurse behind him taking notes on a computer. Yet another screen is mounted high on the wall in front of me so I can see what Dr. Donaldson sees.

What I see is a tiny dot on the screen pulsating incredibly quickly and rhythmically. That's the embryo's heartbeat. And it's all in the right spot: the uterus. I feel incredibly relieved. Then Dr. Donaldson starts going all avuncular on me and saying I should realize that there might be "wastage." It takes me a beat or two until I realize he's warning me that it's very early and I could have a miscarriage—only he's got a pet word for it. Geez, how sensitive.

I have a quick visit with Dr. Herb afterward.

"Everything's absolutely fine," he grins.

info

miscarriage

About one in eight confirmed pregnancies ends in miscarriage. It's believed the figure might be one in four of all pregnancies, but many miscarriages occur very early and are mistaken for a period. As you get older your risk increases; you're also more likely to miscarry if you have already had a miscarriage.

The vast majority of all known miscarriages happen in the first trimester. A miscarriage that happens after week 13 is called a late miscarriage. Loss of a baby after about 20 weeks is called a preterm stillbirth.

You may hear a doctor refer to a miscarriage by the medical term *abortion*. As well, when a pregnancy ends in miscarriage because the embryo does not develop, the embryo is often called a *blighted ovum*. These insensitive medical terms do not help your feelings at the time. Feel free to tell the doctor off for being tactless. They should learn that they're hurting somebody's feelings at the worst possible time, even if to them it's just business as usual.

By far the most common symptom of miscarriage is bleeding from the vagina. If this happens, it is important to contact your health care provider immediately. You will need to be ready to describe the color, quantity, and time frame of the bleeding. Light spotting might not be a cause for alarm and the doctor might tell you to rest for a couple of days. A heavy flow could mean the doctor will tell you that you need to go straight to the hospital.

Vaginal bleeding occurs in about a quarter of pregnant women, but most of them go on to have healthy babies.

During or after a miscarriage you may need to have a small operation to make sure the uterus is free of all the tissue that should come out. The operation is known as a D & C (dilatation and curettage), and is performed under local anesthetic in a hospital. Sometimes a medication is used to help empty the uterus. Other times, the uterus will empty on its own. Danger signs include heavy bleeding, severe pain, and fever. Call your doctor's office's emergency phone number or go to the emergency room if any of these develop.

Don't use a tampon for any bleeding during pregnancy, and keep the pad you do use until you have spoken to your obstetrician. And don't have penetrative sex until the bleeding has been checked by the doctor.

I know this sounds a bit gross and depressing but, if you can, keep any clots and tissue from a miscarriage in a clean plastic bag or container, so they can be examined. This can help your obstetrician decide whether the miscarriage is complete.

Possible causes of miscarriage include "nature rejecting a problem with a pregnancy," such as fetal abnormality; exposure to certain chemicals, illnesses, or medications; problems with the uterus, placenta, cervix, sperm, immune system, or egg implantation; and hormonal imbalances.

An *incompetent cervix* (another charming medical term) is sometimes diagnosed when a late miscarriage occurs. It means that the cervix gets overeager and opens too soon. This is the cause of up to a quarter of miscarriages in the second trimester (week 14 until the end of week 26). Previous gynecological surgery or laser treatments, multiple abortions, or multiple miscarriages could increase your risk of this condition—another reason to give your obstetrician your full medical history. A misbehaving cervix can be stitched closed during your next pregnancy until the baby is ready to come out.

After you've had a miscarriage, get all the information you can from your obstetrician—make sure all your questions are answered—and review the possible risk factors that could be avoided or treated in future pregnancies. If you have more than two miscarriages, you'll usually be tested for uterine problems and hormonal imbalances.

Miscarriage is no less distressing because it's common. Friends and family can make things worse by well-meaning but insensitive remarks, such as "Hurry up and have another one," and "You'll soon get over it." It's important to allow yourself time to talk over and mourn the loss with your partner, who may grieve differently from you, causing friction. It can be really helpful to find a support group so you can talk to and hear from people who have been through it.

 Contact your local hospital, doctor, or a grief counseling service and ask to be put in touch with a support group (see Grief and Loss in Help).

your record

Do you know exactly where and when you got pregnant? After a party, on vacation, while recreational boating perhaps? Take a guess!

What date did you find out you were pregnant? What mix of emotions did you experience? If you have a partner, how did you break the news?

what's going on
Your breasts may be bigger and more sensitive, and the nipples and surrounding areolae may have started to look bigger and bumpier. (The little bumps on each areola are officially called Montgomery's tubercles but who cares about Montgomery, whoever he was: little bumps sounds a lot cuter.) You could have continuing nausea and need to pee a lot. Foods may taste different, and you may hate the smell of things you previously liked.

Teeny buds that will grow into legs are appearing on the embryo. Everything continues growing at a cracking pace. The heart is going strong inside a developing chest but the lungs have only just started to form. Embryonic kidneys begin to develop and function (the finished kidneys come later). The head bulge is getting more like the right shape. The chorionic villi are making more and longer tentacles into

WEEK

the uterus. Some books say the embryo is about the size of a almond or an olive ("Shall I compare thee to a cocktail party nibble?"), but we are officially going with a large coffee bean.

DiARY

I couldn't be less interested in sex if my private parts had been packed away in a shoe box in the back of the closet. This will not do. Where is the surge of lascivious sex-kittenry the books promise and the magazines go on about?

Take the special pregnancy issue of this month's *She* magazine, and I quote: "In the middle of your pregnancy, your libido soars. You're not too enormous but you're round enough not to be concerned about maintaining the missionary position in the quest for a flat stomach and no chins. You bounce about with abandon." What crap.

Apart from the fact that the last thing you want to be thinking about when you're having fun is whether he's thinking about your double chin—and anyway what guy is thinking anything except "Yipee!" with a girlie on top of him?—I'd just like to know where these magazine writers get off, telling us how we're going to feel. As if everybody is the same as them—that is, wanders around saying things like "Beige is the new black, essentials this summer include platform pantyliners with a daisy motif, and in the middle of your pregnancy you'll be a sex-crazed fool."

I've been reflecting on Dr. Donaldson at the ultrasound using the appalling word "wastage" to warn me about a possible miscarriage. It must be his regular spiel to everybody. Anyway it has reminded us again not to tell anyone in case something goes wrong. So we've only told Georgie, Jill, Marg 'cause she's already pregnant, Beck because, let's face it, she is my medical adviser and I'll probably need a bit of advice, Amanda, Steve and Pina, Janie, Lucinda, Mary, Juanita, Heather, Col, and Dave. Less than a hundred people, anyway.

Apart from that I might have to tell some people at work so they don't think I've lost my mind. (I go around with this permanent off-the-air expression, which actually indicates I'm talkin' sales figures and thinkin', "Creature inside me! Creature inside me! Size of a Tic Tac. I feel seasick right now and I have to pretend I don't! Bleeeeuuurghhh! I beg your pardon, I appear to have thrown up on your shoes," or simply "I know something YOU don't know.")

We don't want to tell everyone we're expecting and then have to say, "Oh, we lost it," as if we'd been a bit careless in the Safeway parking lot and left the little bundle in the returned carts section by mistake. I heard that one in eight pregnancies ends in miscarriage.

"Oh, no, that's not right," says Beck.

"Thank God I've got you to calm my fears with proper medical facts, Beck," I say.

"I think it's one in five, or maybe even four," she explains helpfully.

So much of pregnancy seems to be about odds. It automatically turns you into a gambler. The statistics mean everything and nothing at the same time. One in four is high, even if some of those are miscarriages you wouldn't know about because they would be just like having a period. And if you do have a miscarriage, your own personal chance was 100 percent. And if you don't have a miscarriage, your individual risk was 0 percent. But you can't help brooding on "one in four" and every other percentage risk they tell you about.

We go to a birthday barbecue with Matt's family—we don't tell. The next night, Matt's college reunion dinner is full of preggo ladies. Matt wants to tell everyone and has to be sternly restrained.

Poor Matt. He's got a seasick, exhausted girlfriend who'd rather stick peas up her nose than have sex, and he's going to be a daddy. I think we're both feeling kind of like it's all been a theory and now it's actually going to happen. Well, actually, it still feels a bit theoretical. Maybe I'm just in denial.

I know intellectually that I'm pregnant, but it just doesn't feel real. I can't tell by looking, and I don't suddenly feel like knitting booties or protecting my offspring with the ferocity of a lioness. I have no more idea about raising a child than I did 6 weeks ago. No sudden illuminated shaft has split the heavens asunder, pierced the top of my noggin, and said in a very deep voice, "You are going to be a mother." Just as well, really. I'd probably wet my pants.

I am very grumpy. Matt has read somewhere that newborn babies look like their father so the father will stick around. I reply that all newborn babies look like the secretary of treasury of the day, and what's that got to do with anything? Matt wonders why hormones would make you grumpy when surely nature intends you to keep the man happy, to protect you. I refrain from saying that being grumpy is a perfectly damn natural reaction, and furthermore it is no doubt serving the important purpose of teaching you that if the man runs off with a sailor, or proves to be a dead dud at hunting and gathering, you can do it all yourself.

After all, most women with one child and a husband feel like they have two children and anyway why is there a mess in that corner and I believe you forgot to take out the garbage again and WHERE'S MY DAMN DINNER?

info

tiredness

One of the symptoms of the first trimester can be an incredibly draining exhaustion—which you can't even complain about because most people don't know that you're pregnant.

Here's the weird thing: In the past, if you've been really tired, you have probably pushed through it. With first-trimester pregnancy tiredness, you find yourself following your feet down the hall and getting into bed. You have turned into a robot. Welcome to reality: your body is now running you, rather than the other way around.

A lot of women who go to work full-time spend the first tri-mester coming home from their job, going straight to bed, waking up and demanding dinner from their housemate(s) or ordering in takeout for themselves, and then going back to bed.

Most women start to feel perkier and less nauseated by week 14 (but the tiredness comes back in the third trimester).

Here are some of the reasons why you may be so tired:

❂ The high levels of progesterone in the system during the first trimester can have a sedative effect.

❂ Your metabolic rate increases 10 to 25 percent to support the developing fetus, and a whole lot of other parts are working overtime, such as your heart.

❂ Your body is putting the development of the fetus first—you are making eyelids and bones and sex organs and lungs and a placenta and stuff so for heaven's sake who WOULDN'T need to lie down with all that going on?

❂ All that extra nighttime peeing means you're not getting the deepest, most restful part of sleep.

❂ Just being nauseated (see Nausea in Week 4) can make you feel exhausted.

Some ways to combat tiredness are:

❂ Win the lottery; quit work; sleep all the time; get a house cleaner, a masseur, and, oh, forget the expense, a personal chef like Oprah's; live in a posh hotel.

❂ Give in to it, don't fight it—your body will win this round anyway, so you may as well not start your life as a mother by being frazzled.

❂ Let your doctor, midwife, or naturopath know the extent of your first-trimester tiredness: a non-constipating iron supplement may work wonders.

◎ Find a storeroom or sickroom where you can nap if work commitments mean long days at the office (some Pregnant Ladies we know used to just Lie Down under their desks)—and don't forget to eat lunch at your desk if you use the lunch hour for a nap.

◎ Nap when you get home if you work away from home.

◎ Nap when you can if you work at home.

◎ Meet friends for lunch or on weekend days rather than at night (smoky bars and nightclubs, and alcohol, are probably making you feel sick at the moment anyway)—you can always come back to daiquiris in a year or so.

◎ Keep one day, or at least an afternoon on the weekend, completely free; several Pregnant Ladies we know spent All Weekend in bed for the first 3 months.

◎ If you have a partner or roommate who has not been pulling their weight in the housework department, renegotiate so they see that doing the tasks/chores is about rights and responsibilities rather than about "helping" you or doing you a favor; alternatively, get used to mess—or both.

◎ If you already have little children, give them away to relatives. Sorry. No. Try to nap when (if) they do.

peeing all the time

Peeing all the time is a very common symptom of pregnancy in the first 13 weeks or so. It's not that you're overexcited, it's just that your uterus is taking up more space, putting pressure on the neighboring organs, including your bladder. Even more congestion is caused by the extra blood vessels and blood flow developing in the pelvis to sustain the placenta and carry the extra weight.

It may be less of a problem in the second trimester because the uterus "pops" outward at the front, making the pelvis temporarily less crowded. But then constant peeing usually comes back in the third trimester when there's a serious space shortage—at which stage it can feel as if your baby is kicking your bladder, or grabbing it, or generally tossing it around and head-butting it.

You still need to drink lots of water during the day to avoid dehydration, but you can try drinking less in the evenings in an attempt to reduce the number of trips to the bathroom during the night. (Experienced moms will grimly inform you that getting up to pee all night long is good training for the interrupted sleep caused by night feeding once the baby is born. I say try not to do it until you have to.)

If you get a burning or stinging sensation when you pee, mention it to your doctor. You may have a urinary tract infection, and your doctor can help you treat it. Cranberry juice can also help.

what's going on You are

continuing to pee more often because your bladder

is being crowded by the uterus. A lot of fancy

hormonal footwork is going on to keep building the placenta.

You might feel nauseated AND constipated: jackpot! You may

be starting to feel tired: your body has a lot to do that is

normally not on the agenda. Your hair may be getting thicker,

and downstairs there may be more vaginal mucus than normal.

Your embryo has become that classic curled shape,

the big fat head with a tail (not a very attractive shape at this

point, and similar to a prawn from space, sure, but we all

have to start somewhere). It's still SO tiny, but it's

about a million times bigger than the fertilized cell

that started moving and shaking 6 weeks ago.

The external bits of the ears now start to be visible,

and the tiny hands are webbed.

DiARY I am having strange, vivid dreams. Last night I dreamt that author Gore Vidal came to afternoon tea and I gave him Animal Crackers on a silver plate and he said, "How perfectly charming."
I was completely furious that Matt woke me up at that precise moment to kiss me good-bye as he went to work.

"But I just gave Gore Vidal an animal cracker!" I said accusingly.

"Yes, dear," he replied, which was probably about the only thing he could have said.

I also dreamt I went to a carnival on a Pacific island with a well-known model who had too much luggage to fit in the helicopter. In the end it didn't matter as our turn on the Ferris wheel was interrupted by an insistent military coup.

Christmas Day. We spend it pretty quietly, knowing that in the twinkling of an inkling we'll be agonizing over whether to come clean about Santa and how to try to teach a rapacious toddler about the spirituality of giving rather than receiving. (Fat chance.)

I've bought Aunt Peg a pair of silk slippers and an expensive handbag. She's bought Matt and me a plastic fly swatter.

Uncle Stan (we've got him a cell phone) presents us with a book he stole from the mobile library, which he doesn't bother to wrap because wrapping paper destroys the environment. Instead he tapes a homemade card to the front of it. And when I say a homemade card, I mean a bit of cardboard from the inside of his girlfriend's packet of pantyhose. (Reuse, recycle, read my lips: my Uncle Stan is a hippie cheapskate.)

Uncle Stan's new girlfriend is 25 years younger than him and has purple dreadlocks and is a total fruitcake. I suspect she drinks hemlock. Her name, allegedly, is Aurelia. We are already calling her "Oh Really" behind her back.

You can't choose your family, I guess. I wonder how our baby will turn out. Maybe just like Stan. Or just like Mom, but I wouldn't know because I can't remember her. At least I have some photos. Will I have more respect for what she went through, or for the way Aunt Peg and Uncle Stan raised me? Will our child inherit Aunt Peg's instinctive morbid dreads? Or Aurelia's purple dreads? Or be influenced by Uncle Stan's habit of saving rubber bands, rolling them into balls, and then trying to sell them to Mormons who come to the door?

Damned nausea. Queasy isn't the word for it. I am nauseated all the time and desperate for it to stop. Whoever called it "morning sickness" was a complete maniac. (I keep involuntarily singing, "Get it in the morning, get it in the evening, get it at suppertime.") Beck thinks it's just too much estrogen in my system and my liver is having trouble clearing it out.

Aurelia would probably say if I were a Pisces I would accept my pregnancy and wouldn't feel sick and that it's all in my mind. At least I've got a mind, I could tell her.

"The HCG hormone almost certainly has something to do with it, but we don't really know what causes it," Dr. Herb said when I asked him about it during my first visit. I seem to have hit upon a non-infuriatingly-patriarchal doctor.

Why do the preggo books just say, "Eat dry crackers before you get out of bed in the morning"? I mean, that's not very informative, is it? They might as well say: "Sacrifice a chicken and study its entrails. An interestingly shaped spleen means you will continue to have nausea until week 13."

Beck says, "Don't worry, nausea means the baby is hanging on in there. If it stopped suddenly THAT would be a worry because it could mean a miscarriage."

Nausea stops suddenly for a whole day. Oh my God.

Nausea starts again. Thank God.

Damned nausea.

I'm also peeing all the time. In some circles this is regarded suspiciously, and one person even starts a rumor that I have such a severe cocaine problem I have to go to the bathroom three times during a dinner party. In other circles you get smug looks from mothers who think they're onto you. And one of the models at work asked if I was bulimic and suggested I try laxatives instead. Oh, dear.

Matt and I take a long walk on the beach and decide we don't want to have a Down's syndrome baby because it's not fair to have a child who might need constant medical intervention yet might not understand why. And we can't take care of our child forever: one day we'll be gone. We decide that we would terminate if we had to. Matt says the decision is ultimately mine and he'll support it. A part of me knows what he means, and I appreciate the sensitivity, but there's a part of me that gets really annoyed and thinks, "I can't make this decision on my own—we'll both have to live with it." Then I worry about whether I'm a selfish cow. It's all very tricky. Beck advises that if it comes to that, we could always say there was a miscarriage so other people who knew about the pregnancy didn't judge our decision to terminate. Sounds like a good idea. The result of all this is we decide I should have a test that estimates my risk of giving birth to a Down's syndrome baby.

We've chosen an interim name so we don't have to say "it" all the time. Cellsie—as in bunch of cells—is what we're calling the embryo-baby-offspring-thingie inside me. We'll have to come up with something else before kindergarten but it'll do for the moment.

cravings

You know how you sometimes crave chocolate or pasta, or maybe red meat, when you're premenstrual? Pregnancy cravings can be similar. Most pregnant women get a craze for one sort of food or another for a short period—usually ice cream or something sugary. You can go through stages, craving steamed veggies, then chocolate, then tropical fruit. (You can also get disgusted by a food that used to be a favorite. This can include strong-smelling foods and green leafy vegetables that are the slightest bit "slimy.") It's best to keep sugary snacks to a minimum as they don't provide real energy and can stack on extra weight you won't need.

You might get a funny taste in your mouth that seems kind of metallic. This is thought to be due to the high level of various hormones in your blood, which can change the taste of your saliva.

constipation

High progesterone levels are relaxing the muscles in your digestive tract, causing intestinal activity to slow down. This means your poo is going on a slower journey than usual, so it loses water and can become hard, causing constipation. (In the third trimester you can experience even worse constipation as your ginormous uterus squashes the bowel.)

Here are some ways to avoid constipation:

⑥ Drink at least 2 quarts of water, spaced out across the day; try some warm water first thing in the morning if it doesn't make you feel nauseated.

⑥ Eat plenty of natural fiber—fresh and lightly cooked root vegetables, fruit, whole-grain breads, high-fiber cereals such as oatmeal, and brown rice. Choose whole foods instead of processed foods whenever possible. If this is a bulkier load of fiber than your body is used to, have smaller meals more often while you adjust. Remember that the more fiber you eat, the more you need to drink.

◎ Get plenty of exercise.

◎ If chemical iron supplements are causing constipation, talk to your doctor or naturopath about an alternative.

◎ Constipation can also come with the added discomfort of bloating and farting. This should disappear when the constipation goes. Too much unprocessed bran, and sometimes too much raw food, which is hard to digest, can cause bloating. Lightly steamed veggies are easier to absorb than hard, completely raw ones.

◎ Don't take any laxative preparation without discussing it first with your doctor—some laxatives, including those that contain senna, can produce violent expulsive actions, causing painful contractions of the bowel, which in turn can upset the uterus next door.

more info on constipation

Your herbalist or naturopath can help you with natural methods of dealing with constipation, especially after the birth.

Women's Trouble: Natural and Medical Solutions by Ruth Trickey and Kaz Cooke (for details see More Info on Eating and Supplements in Week 2).
This book gives many hints about dealing with constipation naturally, including a seed mix you can add to cereals, and drinks that help things along.

WHOM TO TELL? WHEN TO TELL?

Many people wait until the end of the first trimester (after 13 weeks) to publicly announce their pregnancy, when the greatest risk of miscarriage is over. This allows you time to adjust to the idea of being pregnant and to share feelings in private. It also delays the moment when relatives go berserk and can't shut up about it. Once they know, your mother, mother-in-law, father, and father-in-law (not to mention acquaintances) will descend with advice, horror stories, theories, and judgments about your plans to return to work or not return to work. Even totally positive expressions of joy from your extended family can be overwhelming. Maybe you'll want to pick a weekend to break the news so everyone can celebrate together.

Parents often choose not to tell their toddler until the pregnancy is visible because for a little one it seems like an eternity until something interesting happens. (Well, actually, you don't have to be a toddler.)

Work Exactly when you want to tell your employer will depend on your relationship with them and your position within the organization, but they should hear the news from you and not through the office grapevine. Your employer should be advised in writing that you are pregnant and when you plan to start your maternity leave. You might need to include a doctor's note confirming your due date. You might want to give as much notice as possible so your employer can consider how to best cover your job while you are on leave and how you might make a bleary-eyed return. They'll need time to advertise and interview for your position. Many women hide their pregnancy for as long as they can because of possible discrimination. Before you tell your employer, find out your leave rights (see Getting Ready for Pregnancy in Week 1).

▶

Friends with pregnancy troubles You may have a friend who wants to be pregnant but it's not possible for her right now. She may be having trouble conceiving, have had a miscarriage or several miscarriages, or be in the in vitro fertilization (IVF) program. You may even have a friend whose baby died. The news that you are pregnant will be bittersweet for them. Here are a few hints that might make it easier.

● Tell your friend about your pregnancy privately, perhaps in her home when nobody else is around. Although she will be happy for you, she may have a cry because your pregnancy reminds her so much of what she wants for herself. Don't tell other friends about her situation if she wants to maintain privacy.

● Let your friend know that you will answer any questions about your pregnancy, but that you'll try not to talk to her about it all the time, and that she has your full permission to tell you to shut right up if you get obsessed with baby business.

● It might be a good idea to arrange that your friend first visits you and your new baby at home, away from the hospital, when you won't have other visitors. Don't insist that she hold the baby or discourage her. Don't be alarmed if she cries when holding the baby. She will find her own way to deal with it in her own time.

● Don't for heaven's sake tell her to "just relax" and she'll get pregnant, or insist she try some folk remedy you've read about, or suggest that she do whatever you did. She may already know about an infertility support group or counselor. Often available in both urban and rural areas, these services can usually be contacted through community health centers, family planning centers, and the nearest hospital.

your record

Are you feeling queasy? When?

What smells and/or foods make you feel sick?

What are you doing to combat queasiness?

How have you changed your eating habits during pregnancy?

If you're taking supplements, record them here.

what's going on

Your stomach may not be at all preggie-looking yet. As it grows, your center of gravity will change and you will become, well, a person with the grace of a hippopotamus rather than a fruit bat. So this is the time to attend to any handy-type problems around the house—loose carpeting, tricky steps, bits of bathroom that get slippery or dangerous or awkward to maneuver around. And if there's something you need to get at regularly that involves standing on a stepladder or a chair, lower it for the duration.

The embryo's eyelids appear and its body elongates. The internal sex organs are starting to develop into boy and girl bits, but you can't tell the sex from the outside yet. An ultrasound will be able to show the embryo's early movements. The ends of the limbs are looking a bit more like hands and feet but you still couldn't play "This little piggy goes to market" unless you changed the words to "This little webby bit . . ." Birth guru Sheila Kitzinger's fruit alert says the embryo weighs as much as a grape.

in
1
2
3
4
5
6
7
8

DiARY Even though it still seems miles off, I have to make plans for the actual (it's hard to say this out loud), um, you know . . . birth. I picked up a pamphlet advertising the services of independent doulas at Beck's clinic. You could tell they were very modern because the mother on the front cover, holding her minutes-old baby, had a very charming tattoo on her arm.

I have informed Beck she will have to be my doula and I refuse to get a tattoo. Beck has agreed to this cunning plan, and now I have to ask Dr. Herb if an independent doula can come to the delivery. It feels like being a kid and asking if a friend can stay over, like it's his decision and not mine. The doctor is already in charge. Still, best just to check. You don't want any problems on the day.

We're starting to consider the price of childbirth. We'll be out of pocket about $1,000 to Dr. Herb for prenatal visits and the delivery, which is not totally covered by insurance.

I have also made a reservation at a hospital. It's a small private hospital only 10 minutes away that is owned by some religious people. I don't share their religion, but I'll take their private room. All this stuff arrives from the hospital, which I'm supposed to read and fill out.

There's a hospital admittance form that has on it "Diagnosis: confinement." Confinement?! Hello, can we just shuffle on up to the twenty-first century here for a nanosecond? It's a word out of a Jane Austen novel, or some 1950s sitcom, when pregnant bellies were hidden indoors for the last few months so nobody had to be reminded that pregnant women HAVE HAD SEX. Confined, for Christ's sake. It's a wonder the form doesn't say "BYO handcuffs."

The hospital has a lot of patients who believe in circumcising their boy children. If I have a boy, I might have to write "No circumcision" on his forehead until I leave. And if I can hear all the boy babies screaming, I might just check out and stay at the Sheraton. By the look of how little health insurance covers, the Sheraton might be a lot cheaper. Read in a magazine yesterday how Elle Macpherson checked out of the hospital in a day and went to stay in a luxury New York hotel. Lucky girl. Dr. Herb reminds me that the Sheraton is unlikely to check your hemorrhoids, but I guess you could always try room service.

The list of things we're instructed to bring to the hospital on Cellsie's birthday is more mystifying the longer I look at it. "Underclothes including underpants and nursing bras." Well, what other kinds of underclothes are there? Do people usually bring flounced petticoats and lace teddies? "One to two packages of nursing pads." Oh, dear. Not a clue what they are. Surely nurses can look after their own period needs? "Two packages of super adhesive sanitary pads (maternity sanitary pads such as Whisper)." I can't imagine why they don't have maternity pads called "Ungodly Shrieking". "Whisper" just doesn't seem appropriate somehow.

Then there's a whole list of baby stuff they want you to bring, for which we'll need to borrow a moving van. "Four blankets." Four? What's going to happen to the other three? Does the baby shred them during tantrums? Do they all go on at once? How cold can the kid get? "Baby hat, and booties or socks, and mittens (optional)." Well, I'm glad it's all optional. Because to be honest it hadn't previously occurred to me that a person less than a week old should have a hat and gloves. Stockings, maybe, but let's not go overboard. The kid can develop its own sense of elegant matching accessories when it leaves home and can afford to buy its own formal wear.

Under "What to bring for partner" there is a most unsatisfactorily short list. "Men's night attire please if staying overnight, e.g., sweats, pajamas, robe." (I asked about this, and apparently most of the nurses have seen willies before, but an elderly nurse at the hospital copped an eyeful of a guy's leopard-skin g-string early one morning and took early retirement.)

As Matt has none of the recommended items except sweat pants this could be a bit of a problem. And, anyway, why assume the partner is male? Why should a lesbian partner be forced into men's night attire? It's downright unnatural. And the list of what a partner should bring to the hospital should include: enormous boxes of chocolates, latest magazines, new and attractive clothes, tickets to Paris (springtime), etc. Diamonds would be acceptable.

And a boat with a bowling alley. What am I saying? By the time I give birth we'll have $2.50 between us.

The upshot of reading all this material from the hospital is that you get wildly ahead of yourself. You've still got months and months to go and you're wondering what to pack. Not to mention a few decisions about ambience.

For delivery, the hospital suggests "relaxation music." Not a good start. Relaxation music always makes me very tense. Comedian Mark Little once pointed out it sounded like dolphins playing the piano. Besides, if you gave birth to Enya music, the quietly contemplative ambience might be somewhat offset by the fact that you are screaming the place down and something huge is coming out of your vagina and at least two people you don't even know are watching. And, anyway, if we can subliminally remember birth, why would you want the poor child to forever associate pain, screaming, and fluorescent lights with Enya's latest hits?

Anyway. Further suggestions include camera. Oh, for God's sake, if I want a photo of myself red in the face, grimacing and drooling and shouting I can take a happy snap next time I'm tipsy at a party. Also "essential oils, hard candies, large T-shirt or old nightie, socks, toiletries, book or magazine, etc., T-shirts and shorts or swimwear for partner if desired." I have never imagined labor as a scenario in which I am lying back reading *Pride and Prejudice* while Matt does a few laps. It is all very confusing. And at what exact point during labor would one read a book? "The baby's head is crowning!" "Don't bother me now, Mr. Darcy's just going for a swim in the pond."

fig (A):
OBStetRiciaNS
to Avoid

hello
fatty

<u>info</u>

choosing your childbirth place and team

Even though it seems such a long way off, it's time to start asking around and thinking about what sort of birth you'd like, generally, and who you would like to help you through it. And so begins the search for your primary medical birth attendant and a decision on birth alternatives. Remember that if you live a fair way from a major capital city or large regional hospital, you won't have as many options, so it's even more crucial for you to be well informed and well read about what you *can* demand.

Most people these days look for a safe balance between a comfortable environment and the best medical care available. Giving birth on the kitchen floor is a much safer proposition if there's an ambulance minutes away than if you're in a cabin in the middle of the wilderness with only a confused dog and a potato peeler instead of an experienced midwife.

Because birth can become a medical emergency very quickly, the medical advice is usually to have your baby in a birth center or hospital that has a philosophy you like and can provide an atmosphere you'll feel comfy in but also has specialists and equipment on call.

Home-birth advocates say most medical emergencies develop with plenty of warning, and that home is the best place to give birth.

Some birth options are only available if you have a "low-risk" pregnancy. Your pregnancy is considered "high risk" if, for example, you're going to have a multiple birth or you have chronic high blood pressure or a preexisting condition such as diabetes, or you develop a complication during pregnancy.

where?

What you decide will have a bearing not just on the birth, but also on your prenatal care, and often your postnatal care as well. First you need to decide where you want to have your baby. There are three main options—hospital, birth center, or home.

Hospital Most American women choose to have their babies in a hospital. Many hospitals have created birthing rooms where you can remain through labor, delivery, and recovery. Birthing rooms often have a "homey" feel and are quite comfortable, but are also equipped for emergency situations. They are often seen as the result of hospitals responding to public demand—a safer option than giving birth on a couch at home and a more pleasant and natural option than giving birth on a gurney under klieg lights in a room that smells like industrial-strength Lysol. But "There's much more to a birth room than a double bed and a potted plant," according to one midwife, who warns that some hospital birthing rooms look inviting but have the same hospital attitudes that women are often trying to avoid. You should check that the hospital has staff onsite at all times who can perform a cesarean section in an emergency. Some hospitals require 30 minutes in an emergency situation to call for the anesthesiologist, doctor, and nurses from home.

You can choose to hire an independent, "freelance" midwife or doula—not a hospital employee—who advises you before the birth, stays with you during the birth, and helps you afterward with breastfeeding and other issues. Make sure you check whether the hospital will allow your midwife or doula along with your partner during the labor. Some hospitals are "teaching hospitals," which means medical students and/or residents in obstetrics and gynecology may take part in your care.

Freestanding birth centers These birth centers are not affiliated with a hospital and are not on hospital grounds. Private birth centers are generally staffed by midwives and advocate a "natural child birth" experience. It is important to determine what the plan is if complications arise and you or the baby need hospital care.

Home A home birth is usually attended by midwives. You can choose to have an obstetrician there as well, but your choice will be limited by the fact that very few obstetricians want to be involved in home births, considering them dangerous. You should be transferred to a hospital if it becomes necessary during the delivery. Most health insurance plans will not cover home births, but you may be able to negotiate partial payment for independent midwives and some other services. Check with your insurance company. You should be aware of what will happen if complications occur; whether or not your midwife is certified; and if she has a formal back-up plan agreement with an obstetrician.

who?
The relationship with your obstetrician and midwife who goes with you through pregnancy and beyond is intimate and dependent on trust, mutual respect, and free communication. You'll come to depend on them over a number of months. You will be entrusting them with your life and your child's life. In an ideal situation, they will be equal partners with you in the process.

It's worth spending some time researching and even seeing a couple of candidates before you decide. Recommendations often travel through word of mouth or from your primary doctor. If you feel intimidated, patronized or confused by, or at odds with, an obstetrician or midwife, change to somebody else.

Obstetrician You might prefer a woman obstetrician. Maybe you want a woman obstetrician who has had at least one child herself. Or maybe you don't care if it's a man or a woman as long as the person is fully qualified, pleasant, and easy to talk to (and not called Sparky).

You can ask around for the name of a good one and then get your primary doctor to refer you, or ask your doctor for a recommendation.

Questions you might like to ask an obstetrician on your first visit include:

⑥ Will you be in the country on my due date?

⑥ Who covers for you when you're not on call?

⑥ Under what circumstances are you happy to be contacted during off hours?

⑥ What are your views on pain relief, different labor positions, electronic fetal monitoring, episiotomy, and forceps delivery?

⑥ Under what circumstances would you recommend inducing labor or performing a cesarean?

⑥ What do you consider the roles of the midwife, doctor, mother, and support person or partner to be during the birth?

⑥ How do you feel about following my special wishes for the labor? (We'll get into the birth plans later . . .)

If you're not satisfied with the answers, find another obstetrician.

Tell the obstetrician what sort of birth experience you are hoping for and what sort of patient you are; say, for example, that you like to have clear explanations given to you about why things are done, or that you will be needing extra reassurance because your last pregnancy ended in a miscarriage, or that it's important that you can continue with your alternative health care while seeing the obstetrician, or that you are terrified of the whole idea and thinking of a general anesthetic as well as being out of town at the time or hiding under a rock.

It's important to know that few obstetricians are able to attend the entire labor and birth. They usually pop in and out during labor and are there at the end, for the birth, unless something unusual is happening. So your other support people are very important.

Midwife   There are a few options to choose from.

⊚ You can hire a certified nurse-midwife who'll consult and examine you throughout your pregnancy, attend you at the birth, however long it takes, and advise you on care and feeding during the first weeks of your baby's life. A certified nurse-midwife is a registered nurse who has been certified by the American College of Nurse-Midwives. For women with uncomplicated pregnancies, a certified nurse-midwife is generally qualified for prenatal care and delivery. The midwife can be part of a "shared care" team with your obstetrician or your hospital. They may also attend home births. A midwife will often give you the best continuity of individual care. (Ask the midwife who the "back up" will be in case they can't make it to your birth.) Check with your hospital or birth center whether your midwife has staff priviledges there. Ask your midwife what the back-up system of care will be if there are complications.

⊚ Another option if you desire home birth is a direct-entry midwife. These midwifes are trained only in midwifery and do not have medical or nursing degrees. Some are certified by the North American Registry of Midwives. However, in some states it is illegal for direct-entry midwives to practice.

⊚ Some independent, birth-center, and clinic midwives work in teams. This means a few midwives in rotation might be responsible for your prenatal, delivery, and postnatal care, depending on who is on call or on duty.

 For contact numbers, see under Midwives in Help.

Labor nurse If you're having a hospital birth, the hospital will allocate you a labor nurse. Labor nurses can go "off shift" in the middle of your labor and be replaced by the new labor nurses on duty. Labor nurses implement the obstetrician's orders, monitor the baby and mother, and suggest laboring positions and strategies.

Support person If you have a partner, you'll usually want to have them at the birth. But if your partner isn't willing or able to support you, it's probably better to choose somebody who'll be more useful and supportive at the time. Other common support people are sisters and friends. More rarely, parents are involved, especially mothers. Don't forget that, if you have a long labor, it's better for everyone if your support person gets rest breaks or even a bit of shut-eye. They won't have your endorphins, and you don't want them fainting at the wrong moment (whatever a right moment is).

Some women choose to have a doula attend the birth. A doula has been trained as a labor support person, and she will generally stay with you through your entire labor. This is a new concept, and certification is not standardized. If you decide to hire a doula, interview her and be sure she is comfortable working with other team members at the birth place. Many doulas help with the first few weeks at home, including breastfeeding.

Many people want a record of the event in photos or on video: some even want it shown live on the Internet. It can be hard for somebody to be in charge of support, candy, and multimedia at the same time.

Some people invite a cast of thousands, only to regret it later. Don't forget the people who are actively involved need room to do their work. Some midwives and doctors believe that the more people in the room, the longer the labor. Most women don't want to be distracted by visitors or worried about how their small children are coping with what can be a pretty heavy scene for them.

your record

What kind of prenatal and birth care have you
chosen? How did you find your obstetrician or
midwife? Whom did you choose? Who else will be
on your support team and why?

ultrasound

WEEK

what's going on
You're hungry. Eat. Your body is doing a lot of work and you need more fuel than usual.

The embryo officially becomes a fetus this week. Very few organs are actually working yet, but they're in the right spot. The head is still big in proportion to the rest of the fetus. The nostrils and tear ducts are finished. (If anybody asks why you're tired, just say you've been making eyebrows all night long.) Around about now the little tail will "disappear" as the rest of the fetus grows. The limbs get longer; the arms can bend; hands and feet can touch each other; and toes and fingers lose their webbing and become fully separated. Sheila Kitzinger's never-ending supply of fruit comparisons says your uterus is now the size of an orange. Weight: about $1/4$ ounce.

Average approximate fetus length this week from head to butt

in
1
2
3
4
5
6
7
8

Diary I'm not sure but I think some of my wrinkles—sorry, I mean character lines—are less obvious. This is because my body is making extra collagen and all that stuff the cosmetics companies would probably kill us pregnant women for if they knew how to get it out of us.

Most of my daily thoughts consist only of the following mantra: "I have no interest in food, I cannot cook, I must lie down, I need to watch crap on television, would you get a load of Ricki Lake's hairdo. Help me. I can't get off the couch." It's all just too, too exhausting. If only I were the sort of person with four servants and a heart-shaped box of chocolates and a four-poster bed with a quilted-satin duvet cover, it would probably all look quite glamorous. I could have a negligee and a peignoir, and other French words for "jammies."

I go for the nuchal fold ultrasound. This is an ultrasound that looks for a thickening at the back of the baby's neck, which is an indicator of Down's syndrome. For some reason everyone thought I might be 11 weeks pregnant but it's actually only about 10 according to the ultrasound operator, Dr. Donaldson. Which means it's too early to see much and I'll have to come back again.

It was kind of disappointing not to get a definitive answer about the nuchal fold thing, but I'm happy that somebody else is as bad at math as me. Matt comes for a look. There's Cellsie on the screen, waving its little bits.

"There's your baby," says Dr. Donaldson.

"It's not, it's a beetle," I retort, looking at an insecty shape stuck on its back and wiggling a lot of little legs in the air.

"Look, it's waving," he says, pointing out a head, two arms, and two legs.

The head seems to turn toward us, like something out of an alien movie.

"Oh fuck, that's too weird," I say and nobody answers.

It occurs to me that you're not supposed to say "fuck" during an ultrasound. Repeat after me: Mommies ought not to say "fuck." Sigh. So much to learn.

The creature on the screen looks like any sort of fetus. It could grow into a lizard, or a lap-dance club owner, or something equally

hideous. And even though inside me it's actually only about
1 1/2 inches long, on the screen it looks as long as an adult hand.
This is very disconcerting. Makes it seem more advanced and less
human at the same time.

Suddenly the heartbeat monitor at the bottom of the screen
shows an up-and-downie, mountain-shaped graph running along
like something out of *ER*—and the sound! Like a Latin techno beat!
The fastest heartbeat I have ever heard. Looking closer, we can see
the heart actually beating inside the lizardy thing. I begin to feel
quite fond of it.

"That's not my heartbeat, is it?" I ask. "Because if it is, I think
I'm having a heart attack."

Dr. Donaldson doesn't know why fetal heartbeats are so fast,
but he says it's quite normal. Everything is normal. Size, normal.
Shape, normal. All bits present so far. Normal. Normal, normal,
normal.

Normal? I want to sneer. I've spent my whole life running away
from normal. I don't DO normal. I refuse to live in the suburbs.
I want to be special, I want to be interesting, I want . . . Okay, it's
kind of reassuring that everything's normal. I'll admit it. You don't
want to hear an ultrasound operator saying "What the . . . ?"
"That can't BE!" or "Holy catfish! I've never seen that before. Do
you mind if I call some friends to come over and have a look?."

(Matt confesses afterwards that he checked out the electronic
equipment and was watching the $5,000 monitor while I was
watching the $1,000 monitor. He promises to point out the
superior hardware next time we go.)

Dr. Donaldson gives us a speech about how we shouldn't do
any further tests unless the nuchal fold ultrasound shows a possible
problem. He says once you start getting tests done they will often
give false positive results, and then you just have more tests. He
says our chances of having a Down's syndrome baby are less than
the chances of losing a healthy pregnancy because one of the
tests—amniocentesis (often called "amnio")—may trigger a
miscarriage. More statistics. There's a 1 in 500 chance of
Down's syndrome and a 1 in 200 chance of the test causing a
miscarriage.

Another consultation with Dr. Herb, clutching the normalnormalnormal ultrasound report in my hand. There's got to be a more civilized way of arriving at the doctor's than putting your jar of pee on the counter and then trotting off to the scales and shouting out to the doctor's assistant, "One-hundred-seventy pounds, Lorraine, but 20 pounds of that must be these hiking socks I'm wearing."

Lorraine, of course, invariably calls across the waiting room, "HOW much do you weigh, again?" or "IS THIS YOUR PEE, MADELINE?"

I imagine we're now going live through the hospital's public address system: "Madeline Harridan is 170 pounds, Madeline Harridan is 170 pounds, code red." All heads turn. "Look, Lorraine, just write down: 'Has entered bovine stage. When she walks, bass drum and tuba music plays. Was mistaken for a sea cow off the beach early this morning.'"

I further distinguish myself once I get into Dr. Herb's room by whipping off my skirt and undies when he just wants to feel my tummy and measure the fundus.

The man obviously thinks I'm some kind of crazed exhibitionist who enjoys lying on couches naked from the waist down except for boots, while her boyfriend sits in the corner reading a pamphlet.

Well, maybe I am. What's it to ya?

I wonder what a fundus is? Oh. It's the top of the uterus.

Dr. Herb expands on the statistics of various risks. It leaves my brain in a whirl of confusing math, so it seems best to just wait and see what's on the next ultrasound.

I have started to wrestle with constipation: I decide to adopt Beck's secret seed-breakfast method. Every time I get constipated I get at least one pimple, probably two. But after a day or two of crushed mixed seeds on my muesli, I'm running like a train again and zit free.

info

chromosomes and genes

At conception the egg and sperm join to make a single cell. This one cell, combining twenty-three chromosomes supplied by the egg and twenty-three from the sperm, contains the entire genetic blueprint for your child. At that moment, your baby's genetic destiny is decided: what sex it will be; how tall it will be; how much natural musical or sporting talent it will have; what color skin, hair, and eyes; what shape it will become after puberty; and maybe what kind of illnesses it will be prone to.

Even though its genetic inheritance comes equally from both parents, a baby will not be an exact 50:50 mix of both parents' characteristics. It may end up with red hair that has skipped a generation, or with a skin color that is far more Dad than Mom, or vice versa. Your child may look not much like either parent, but more like long-lost Great-Aunt Minnie. Some families have genes that always seem to win out, such as a distinctive family nose or a particular build.

Your baby will eventually have millions of cells. The forty-six chromosomes inside the nucleus of each cell are made up of two chains of your genetic code, called DNA (deoxyribonucleic acid), which control the growth and functioning of the baby. The chromosomes contain thousands of genes, which determine the physical and intellectual characteristics.

problems with chromosomes and genes

The term "genetic disorder" refers to changes in the genetic code—like a typing error—that occurred in the formation of the genes and chromosomes in a particular baby, as well as to medical conditions or health problems that are inherited through the family.

Some inherited genetic diseases such as cystic fibrosis happen when both parents carry a recessive gene that can cause a problem. This gene doesn't affect either of the parents, but when the two potential problem genes are combined the fetus is affected. Other problems such as hemophilia (in boys) may be "activated" only if the baby is of a certain sex. Some genetic disorders are linked to geographic regions or ethnic groups. Sickle-cell anemia is the most common genetic disease in people of African descent, for example.

Down's syndrome is a genetic condition with a high profile. The most common cause of intellectual disability, it affects about 1 in 800 to 1,000 pregnancies. It is also known as trisomy 21. Because of an accident during the division of cells when still an embryo, the fetus has three copies of chromosome 21 instead of the usual two. A Down's syndrome baby (and adult) will be mentally disabled, will have characteristic facial differences (especially a distinctive eyelid shape), a stocky stature, and loose muscle tone, and may also suffer from medical problems, such as heart abnormalities, that need corrective surgery.

The incidence of Down's syndrome increases dramatically in the fetuses of older women. The ratios are:

21-year-old women—1 in 1,520 pregnancies
35-year-old women—1 in 355 pregnancies
40-year-old women—1 in 90 pregnancies
43-year-old women—1 in 40 pregnancies

genetic counseling

Your hospital or your obstetrician can refer you to a genetic counselor for any of the following reasons, but it is not automatic. If you have any worries you may need to bring up the subject.

◎ You've had a diagnostic test confirming a chromosomal abnormality.

◎ You've had miscarriages.

◎ You or your partner has a family history of inherited physical or psychiatric disease.

◎ Blood tests have indicated a partner carries a genetic disorder.

◎ You've already had a baby with a chromosomal or genetic abnormality.

◎ You've had a baby who died before or shortly after it was born.

◎ You or your partner or a member of either family was born with an abnormality caused by a genetic problem that was not inherited through the family—this is known as a congenital abnormality.

◎ You and your partner are related (cousins, for example).

◎ You will be 35 or older at the time of the birth.

Genetic counselors can accurately assess your risk of having a baby with a hereditary disorder. If you have already had a child with a disorder, they may be able to predict your chances of it happening again. They can tell you if you carry genes that cause certain disorders and very often reassure you that the chances of a problem are very low. The techniques used to arrive at this information can include blood tests, genetic analysis, and examination of both families' medical history. So of course it will always be a bonus if you have access to family histories on both sides. If you don't have access because you don't know who the father is or he is uncooperative, you probably don't need to worry at all. Genetic problems are very rare.

more info on gene and chromosome problems

There are support and info groups for various genetic disorders. Check the phone listings for your area or call the genetic counselor at the biggest hospital in your area.

Which Tests for My Unborn Baby? by Lachlan de Crespigny and Rhonda Dredge, Oxford University Press, Oxford, England, 1996.

An informative book that explains risks, tests, results, and the decision-making process during what could be your most confusing moments. Compassionate case histories add to the nonjudgmental tone.

your record

If the baby's dad is on the scene, how does he seem to
be reacting? You might like to get him to write down
his thoughts here, or you could put your hair in a bun
and take dictation and then take all your clothes off
and . . . excuse me.

Average approximate fetus length this week from head to butt

1

2

3

4

5

6

7

8

what's going on Nausea

should start to settle down from now on.

Hurrah.

Outside influences, such as certain drugs

and chemicals, could have damaged the fetus

while it was still forming; the dangers are still there

after week 10 but are no longer so acute.

(This does not mean you can chug the vodka.)

The placenta is continuing to get

bigger, keeping pace with what the

fetus needs. The heart is completely

formed and pumping away. The ear

and hearing structures are nearly

finished and ready to grow. Your fetus is looking

a lot more like a tiny human with a big

head, short limbs, and not much fashion sense.

(In fact, about now the head is almost half the size

of the whole fetus.) Weight: about $1/3$ ounce.

WEEK 11

oops

INADVISABLE ACROBATIC DANCING

DiARY I've been lent a lot of baby-care books for the duration. One is Aunt Peg's decrepit second-hand copy of Dr. Spock from approximately the Jurassic period, which she immediately borrowed after Mom died to work out what she and Uncle Stan should do with this small creature (me) suddenly on their doorstep.

I took a look at the modern pregnancy and child-care books, but I discovered most of them are absolutely terrible. For one thing, they're always banging on about husbands as if every pregnant woman had to have one. Mind you, it's not just insulting to the single mother-to-be. The guys don't come out of it well either. One book actually recommends that you teach your husband to make his own breakfast before you go to the hospital, say by week 32 to be sure. If a guy doesn't know how to make his own breakfast, I say you're better off without him.

It's kind of comforting that even the experts disagree—this means you don't have to get worried if you're not at exactly the stage a book reckons you should be. On almost every major yardstick I'm not. And quite frankly I don't expect to have a multiple orgasm the first time I breastfeed.

Even some of the good books have the most absurd photographs to enliven their pages. Under the section on nutrition or appetite there is usually a photograph of a woman with a plate of food, in case you have forgotten what a plate of food looks like.

And I don't wish to be rude, but I'd like all the people who have done illustrations for pregnancy books rounded up and killed. They can't be allowed to go on. Who ARE all these women in the illustrations, pale-as-pastry, frumpy, with disgusting haircuts, wearing duvet covers? And who are these husbands with gigantic sideburns looking manfully into the distance? They are the line-drawing equivalents of knitting-pattern photos from the 1970s. With captions like "A new father can bottle-feed a baby." Yes, and given half a chance he can tie his own shoelaces, and all.

One book has four dirty drawings of bright-pink couples "making love" during pregnancy, in different positions. In the first position they look bored. In the second position they look like they've had a lobotomy. In the third they look really smug, and in

the fourth, I don't know how this is quite conveyed, but I'm
pretty sure they were singing "Michael Row the Boat Ashore."
(This could be dangerous. If you don't know by now that it's
possible to have sex from behind, a line drawing is going to send
you into shock.)

Another book, called *A Child Is Born*, has graphic photos of the
fetus in the uterus. It's disgusting. Matt reads it every night. He's
fascinated by the pictures. They make me want to projectile vomit.

"Look, that's what Cellsie looks like now."

I scream and hide under the sheets. "That looks like a prawn
made of snot!"

"But it's amazing. Look at this one—this is what it'll look like
next week."

Great. A portion of especially dumb plankton, with eyes like
ball bearings. I cannot relate to this. It is a greater test of maternal
instincts than anyone should have to undergo. Nobody could love
a snot prawn. How can I bond with a crustacean?

There really is too much information in these books, and yet
not enough. For example, "Acrobatic dancing is, of course, unwise
at any stage during pregnancy." How acrobatic? Are we talking
those circus girls who can put their head up their own butt? Do we
refer here to the sort of wafty crap, Stevie-Nicks-type hippie
dancing while waving shawls? Which is surely ultimately more
offensive and therefore more dangerous than the lesser-known
acrobatic dancing.

And personally I cannot take anybody seriously who uses the
word "brassiere" in a complete sentence. Especially if the sentence
is "The advantage of having a well-made and properly fitted
brassiere cannot be emphasized too strongly." Certainly not,
Mrs. Shelf-Bosom. Emphasize away.

One of the books, by Miriam Stoppard, has an entire section
devoted to how to wear makeup during pregnancy (on your face, I
presume). Anyway, there are handy hints such as how to cover up
dark circles under the eyes, and camouflage puffiness by shading a
little brown blush subtly beneath the jawbone and on either side
of the neck. Look, this might work if you are standing still, being
professionally lit and photographed, but if you're walking around

like a normal human being, no amount of brown blush on your neck is going to disguise the fact that you're a bit puffy.

You would be better off constantly introducing yourself to people by saying, "Hello, I'm a bit puffy. It's because I'm pregnant and a big fat baby is going to come out of my vagina," and getting on with things. I can guarantee nobody will mention any puffiness after that. Not to your face, anyway. Here's a great pregnancy makeup hint: "To draw attention away from your jawline, try using a blush at the temples so that your eyes become the focus." Or, say, wear a hat with a rotating stuffed zebra leg on it.

info

screening and diagnostic tests

There are lots of screening and diagnostic tests that will give you an idea of how your baby is developing, although not all of them are 100 percent accurate.

A screening test is one that assesses your risk (against the average risk) of carrying a baby who has certain abnormalities. A positive screening-test result does NOT mean the baby has an abnormality. In fact, chances are very much in your favor that the baby is perfectly fine, but the result means that a further test is offered to you, a diagnostic test.

Diagnostic tests, such as amniocentesis and CVS (see below), can provide you with a definite answer about whether your baby has a specific abnormality. Ultrasound tests are also used, but they're not a fail-safe way of detecting problems. For the best chance of useful results, an ultrasound test must be conducted by a specialist operator.

More than 95 percent of women having prenatal tests will have babies with no abnormality at all.

routine ultrasound

An ultrasound examination bounces high-frequency sound waves into your body to create an image of the fetus and your internal organs on a computer screen. You lie on your back while an ultrasound technician or obstetrician performs the test. A small object a bit like a computer mouse will be run over the top of your tummy, after some gel has been spread on it; or, if the test is done before twelve weeks of pregnancy, a "probe" is put into your vagina. Luckily the probe is only about the size of a large pen. Ultrasounds don't hurt, and these days you may not have to have a full bladder.

An ultrasound is usually offered to you at about 19–21 weeks. It's a great chance to see your fetus on screen for the first time—so bring your partner, or a friend who might get a kick out of it. If you're lucky, the fetus will give you a wave. It can be quite an emotional moment seeing your fetus for the first time; be prepared to get misty eyed.

The operator will compile a report for your obstetrician. The ultrasound can confirm an estimation of how advanced your pregnancy is (give or take a few days); catch sight of twins or multiple babies; and locate the position of your placenta (if it's lying low, another ultrasound will be done later in the pregnancy to see if placenta previa has developed—that's when the placenta grows over or very close to the cervix). The ultrasound will show any uterine growths, such as fibroids. Most fibroids are harmless and don't get in the way of anything—you wouldn't even know you had them unless you'd had the ultrasound.

An ultrasound allows the operator to measure and observe limbs and organs; it also shows the baby's gender (it's about 98 percent accurate, but sometimes the position of the fetus can make identification difficult). If you don't want to know the sex of the baby you should let the operator know; otherwise they're likely to blurt out something like "It's a girlie!" or "Look out, there's a big willy."

A specialist ultrasound operator can usually identify certain fetal abnormalities such as spina bifida, cleft palate, and misshapen feet by using measurements and observation.

Digital technology has made it possible now to have a three-dimensional ultrasound. Distributors of this technology say it is better than the routine ultrasound at picking up some abnormalities early on, but the scientific research has not confirmed this.

nuchal fold ultrasound

You may be offered, or you can request, an ultrasound at 11–12 weeks that is sometimes called the nuchal fold, or nuchal translucency, test. The operator gets a good image of your fetus's neck on the screen and measures the skin layer at the back of the neck. The thicker this layer is, the greater the chance the baby will have Down's syndrome. (This test picks up about 80 percent of Down's syndrome cases it surveys.) If the neck swelling is there, you will be offered a more accurate diagnostic test—amniocentesis or CVS (see below)—which can tell you whether or not your baby has Down's syndrome.

expanded alpha-fetoprotein or triple screen test

Your doctor will probably suggest a blood test, carried out between 16–18 weeks, to find out if you have an increased risk of Down's syndrome or neural tube defects such as spina bifida. A small amount of blood is taken from your arm and sent off to a laboratory. The result comes back within a week as either "low risk" or "increased risk," often expressed as a statistic (a 1 in 30,000 chance, 1 in 100, and so on). Nineteen out of twenty women tested will have a "low risk" result.

An "increased risk" result does *not* automatically mean your baby has the conditions tested for, but it does mean you'll probably be offered a further diagnostic test: an ultrasound, CVS, or amniocentesis. (Most "increased risk" women will be found to be carrying a healthy baby. Unfortunately this means you often sweat on a "1 in 30" result for two weeks until you get the all clear.) The blood test works by measuring levels of substances in the blood including the hormone HCG, the estrogen called estriol, and a protein called alpha-fetoprotein. An early blood test, done between 9–12 weeks, can be interpreted with the nuchal fold test to predict almost 90 percent of Down's syndrome cases.

amniocentesis and CVS

Some diagnostic tests are usually recommended if you're 35 or older at the time of birth, you have a family history of Down's syndrome or spina bifida, you've had a fetus with a neural tube defect in a previous pregnancy, you've had an "increased risk" blood test result, or you've had an inkling from the ultrasound that your fetus may be at greater risk.

The two main diagnostic tests are amniocentesis (known as "amnio") and CVS (chorionic villus sampling, but it's almost always just called CVS). These are both invasive tests that slightly increase your existing risk of miscarriage—amnio by half of 1 percent and CVS by 1 percent when carried out by experienced, specialist practitioners.

It's this risk that makes the tests optional rather than a routine for every pregnancy. You will be weighing up a statistical risk—the chance of discovering a defect versus the chance of causing the miscarriage of a healthy fetus. Help in making that decision is available from your obstetrician or hospital prenatal clinic.

Operators' risk rates can vary enormously, so insist that your obstetrician refer you to a place where the procedure is performed by experienced specialists (this might mean you need to travel to your nearest large city), and ask the obstetrician about the risk rate of the particular person who will be performing your procedure.

Amniocentesis is used to test for Down's syndrome and other chromosomal disorders, neural tube defects such as spina bifida, and other genetic conditions. The test is carried out at about 16 weeks. It involves you lying very still, while the technician uses an ultrasound to see exactly where the fetus is inside the amniotic sac. The doctor will then insert a needle through your abdomen and into the uterus but not near the fetus. The needle draws in a small amount of amniotic fluid, which contains cells from the fetus. It is these cells that can give a definitive answer to questions about chromosomes.

CVS is used to test for most of the same conditions as amnio, but it cannot test for spina bifida. The test is often done earlier than amnio and can be done at any time after about 11 weeks. The doctor operates in much the same way as with amnio but takes a needle sample of tissue from the chorion—the name for the placenta in its early, growing phase. The needle can go in either through the abdomen or through the vagina.

Both tests are usually considered to be uncomfortable rather than painful, although it's no fun having a big needle put into you near your fetus; besides, you may be worried about the result. It's good to have someone come with you to the procedure who can then take you home, where you should lie down for the day, or even two, depending on the advice of your obstetrician. Sexual activity should be put on hold for a few days.

Results for both tests take up to 3 weeks. Because CVS can give a result earlier in the pregnancy than amnio, it's often helpful if you have to decide whether to discontinue a pregnancy involving a fetus with an abnormality. It is easier emotionally and physically to terminate a pregnancy as early as possible. Most people do decide to terminate a fetus with a severe abnormality, but some would not do this whatever the circumstances.

Decisions about terminations are always difficult, even if you're sure you've made the right choice. Take as much time as possible to thoroughly work through and feel comfortable with the decision. Nondirective counseling will be available to you (help to understand and process the issues, without any urging in a particular direction); it can also be useful in resolving any differences of opinion between you and your partner.

Some elements to consider are the nature and severity of the diagnosed condition, the likely survival or quality of life of the baby after birth, any ethical and religious aspects, your willingness and ability to deal with the baby's condition, and the likely impact on members of your family such as other children.

If your obstetrician does not wish to terminate the pregnancy once you have decided you want to, see another one or go to a family planning clinic (see Family Planning Clinics in Help for contact numbers). If your obstetrician strongly advises you to terminate, and you are unsure or don't want to, the same altern-atives apply.

Even if for religious or ethical reasons you would not consider terminating your pregnancy, these tests can help you and your family to prepare in both an emotional and practical sense for the birth requirements and care of a special-needs baby, or for the possibility of a miscarriage.

more info on tests and beyond

Which Tests for My Unborn Baby? Ultrasound and Other Prenatal Tests by Lachlan de Crespigny with Rhonda Dredge, Oxford University Press, Melbourne, 1998. Written by an obstetrician and a journalist specializing in genetics, this is a surprisingly easy to follow, up-to-date explanation of the hows and whys of ultrasound, CVS, amnio, and fetal abnormalities, and it also provides a wrap-up of less common testing procedures.

Your nearest family planning clinic, hospital maternity ward, or obstetrician will have staff and counselors to help you, and pamphlets or booklets you can read on specific issues. There are support groups for parents of babies and children with special needs. Your doctor or nearest hospital should be able to help you get in touch.

Grief counselors can help with anything from a decision to ter-minate or miscarriage to dealing with a special-needs baby.

See also Grief and Loss, and Babies' Health Problems, in Help.

your record

What tests have you decided to have?

How do you feel about waiting for results?

If you had an ultrasound, what was it like? What could you see? You can paste in any ultrasound photos here.

1

2

3

4

5

6

7

8

what's going on This is often the first time

you'll visit the obstetrician. Don't forget beforehand to write

down questions for the obstetrician as they occur to you. You

may be feeling very tired—after all, you're not just a fascinating,

sophisticated minx any more, you're a walking host organ.

Inside, your fetus looks more like a baby but with the

head still bent forward. The face has a human profile and

the jaw hides twenty developing tooth buds. Muscles are

growing and increasing the movement of the fetus, but you still

can't feel it because it has plenty of room to slosh about in the

amniotic fluid without touching the sides. As the placenta has

been doing since week 5, it is routinely sending oxygen and

nutrients down the vein of the umbilical cord, and taking

away waste such as fetal pee, which travels back up

the two arteries in the cord. Weight: about 3/4 ounce.

DiARY

For some reason my sense of smell has become really acute. I can only wear men's aftershaves. Any even slightly girlie, florally scents make me go bleuuuergh. God help me if I get stuck in an elevator at a department store.

Finally I get to have the real nuchal fold ultrasound. This time Dr. Donaldson pokes Cellsie around to get it in the right position by pushing hard on my tummy, and I really don't feel good about this. All the measurements are fine, he says, and so he would advise against me having further, invasive tests. Again we are at the whim of statistics, reminded that the test picks up 80 percent of Down's syndrome cases. For a wild math-phobic moment I think this means we have a 20 percent chance of having a Down's syndrome baby, but of course it doesn't mean that at all.

We leave, and I surprise myself by bursting into tears. For some reason I feel great indignation at Cellsie being unceremoniously poked to get him or her into a better position. I guess the baby must be starting to feel more real. I didn't expect to feel protective of my little space prawn.

We're close to the magic, don't-have-to-be-so-scared-about-miscarriages point, and we decide to tell everybody we haven't told. Matt's parents are thrilled and send us a lovely fax from Canada, where they are on assignment investigating a rare fungus up some mountain. Aunt Peg is very happy, I think, but it's hard to tell. Aunt Peg cries no matter what happens.

Uncle Stan seems very happy, but then he's cheered up immensely since the initial shock when Aunt Peg changed the locks after the Mandii the Magnificent incident 11 years ago. Sure it took him 10 years, but he's certainly making out in the jollies department. He seems seriously avuncular about the idea of a grandniece or nephew.

He makes the same joke he does every 2 months about being glad we're not getting married so he doesn't have to pay for it. Anyway, he continues, the State should have nothing to do with religion, which is why Stan's a Pagan. He likes to write it in purple ink on his census form every 10 years. Actually I think he's decided to be a Pagan because at Pagan Rituals you get to meet a lot of mature-age ladies who wear shawls, listen to Fleetwood Mac, and agree to have Sex with Stan.

As Aunt Peg snorts: "Pagan, my ass. He's a Christian." Even though she hasn't been to a church, except for a wedding, in 30 years, as far as Aunt Peg is concerned everyone is Christian except "foreigners." (When I told her I was happily going to have the baby in a Jewish hospital because it was the closest, she had to lie down.)

At the news of our impending bundle of joie de vivre, Stan's girlfriend Aurelia shrieks, throws herself off her stilettoes onto Matt, gets coral-colored lipstick in his eyebrows and his ears (she's thorough), and expresses the opinion that a few good thumps never hurt anyone and she hopes we won't be the type to coddle the little bastard. I repress the urgent desire to reassure her that we'll start whacking the living daylights out of it as soon as we see its head coming out, but I find it harder than usual to be jocular about child abuse in my present state. Guess it's those pesky "baby hormones" the books blame everything on.

Aurelia demands that Uncle Stan take her to the bar to celebrate. Uncle Stan departs, saying he's very happy for us but he's never changed a diaper in his life and he doesn't intend to start now, damn it. I think everyone has made their position clear. Five minutes later Uncle Stan comes back to get Aurelia's gold Glo-mesh cigarette case.

"Your mother would have loved this," he whispers.

I get tears in my eyes. I've always missed her, but I think I'll feel it more when the baby comes.

Apparently the minute she got there, Aurelia announced my pregnancy to the bar, the ladies' lounge, and the men's urinal, as well as to a guy called Scott who was rewiring a pinball machine.

Matt's cousin Annie, mother of six, which is a truly appalling prospect, the one who spent years before the pregnancy asking when I was going to get pregnant and then, when told to knock it off, asked everyone else in the family every time she saw them, is continuing to be insufferable. She announces loudly and frequently, "I *knew* you were pregnant!" and has taken to poking me in the stomach and squeezing me on the arm as if she's about to buy me as a Shetland pony for one of her children. "Mmm," she says each time. "Yes, you're definitely pregnant!" "No, I just said I was for something to do, you idiot," I feel like saying. Or "Yes, I had an inkling. I feel pregnant and the hormone tests say I'm pregnant and I've seen the fetus on ultrasound."

Other immediate reactions to "I'm pregnant" have included:

"You'll never get rid of them!" (60-year-old woman)

"That's wonderful!" (all the nice people I know)

"Your life is over!" (Miss Francine, my beautician)

Complete silence and choking sound. (my boss)

One of my clients buying the latest line wants me to commit to a fashion conference 4 hours away by plane, in September. Cellsie will be 4 weeks old. "It will only be for a day and a half," he says. "You'll be dying to get out and about by then, and reclaim your identity. I mean, I know when we had kids it satisfied my creative urges for a while, but then you really need to reclaim your own space." Lordy. What a dork.

Another visit to Dr. Herb so he can check out the ultrasound results, and me. Wait in the waiting room while he delivers somebody else's baby. (Well, one can hardly complain about *that* as an excuse for being late, can one?) The woman next to me has a small child she speaks to in a Very Loud Voice. She is Extremely Annoying. The child looks at pictures in a book.

"Here's Daddy," he says, pointing to a man.

"That's not *our* daddy," she bellows, cheerfully.

Our daddy! "Ma'am," I feel like saying, "he is the child's daddy. He is not your daddy." I ponder the whole spooky idea of calling your sexual partner Mommy or Daddy.

Finally I get to see Dr. Herb. He gives the old tummy a bit of a poke and a feel (this is called palpation apparently) and seems pleased with the progress.

"It's definitely growing."

Despite the obviousness of this banality I am absurdly pleased. He smiles.

"Everything's going as well as could be expected. Couldn't be better." I beam. Oh hurrah. I feel like I've received a gold star and an elephant stamp on my homework.

"By the way, I had some reeeeally alcoholic punch at a party when I was already pregnant," I 'fess up.

"How much?" asks Herb.

"About two glasses. Erm. Maybe three. Four, tops."

"It's very unlikely to do any harm at all."

Phew.

I have written down three questions: Can Beck be the doula? (Yes.) Is the hospital set up for any emergency, and will he perform a cesarean if it's needed? (Yes.) And what books does he recommend? (Janet Balaskas's *Active Birth*.) I think it's interesting that, of all the books on pregnancy and child-wrangling, he has chosen one about birth, but I realize afterward that he must have thought I MEANT just books on childbirth because I had asked about the hospital facilities. You have to be so specific. They see so many women in a day. God knows how many sailor collars on circus-tent dresses the poor man has had to endure in his lifetime.

Aunt Peg is driving me insane. She has been depressed since 1957, but she carries about her the air of a wounded martyr delivering vital messages to the front. Unfortunately, now she knows I'm pregnant, she has decided the front is me and the messages must be as tragic as possible. Aunt Peg always has a horrendous story to tell, usually about some dreadful thing that has happened to a small child: left in the wilderness, flung from a train, attacked by feral guinea pigs—you name it, Aunt Peg can tell you the long version.

"I'm not congratulating Matt yet, dear," she announces on the doorstep instead of saying hello, "in case something goes wrong."

Tact and optimism are strangers to our Peg. After a few other pleasantries (babies who have been abused, small children murdered by their estranged parents, the children of women who drink too much in pregnancy), she bursts into tears—just as I am about to shovel her into the gutter and get to work.

"Oh, poor little thing!" she sobs.

I am bewildered. "Who?"

"Kimberley."

"Kimberley?" I reply, mystified. The only Kimberley I know is a strapping second cousin of 42 years, who lives in ignorant bliss with her idiot husband and five children.

"Yes," sobs Aunt Peg, who's related to this person by marriage. "Her mother lifted a stone block when she was 6 months and 17 days pregnant, and Kimberley came the next day."

"But Kimberley is perfectly fine, apart from being a complete idiot," I reply.

Aunt Peg looks at me accusingly. "You're not lifting anything, are you?"

She leaves, after pressing some packets of herbs into my hands, neatly labelled with their names.

"Make yourself some tea with these, dear, they're very natural," she confides.

No way. After she goes I call Beck for the herb inside story, and sure enough, one of the herbs is an abortifacient, which means it could abort or deform a developing fetus. Now I have to call Aunt Peg and tell her to stop being an amateur herbalist around town before somebody breaks out in hives, loses their hair, or kicks the bucket. (What is it about pregnancy that brings out the amateur doctor or herbalist in people?)

"Your Aunt Peg," says Matt that night, "is nuts. It probably runs in the family."

info

pregnancy hormones

Every time you mention a symptom of pregnancy—from bigger breasts, to being grumpy, to wanting an ice cream, to feeling unspecific morbid dread, to wanting to stand on the roof and shriek—somebody will say in tones of enormously ponderous knowledge, "It's the pregnancy hormones." Well, what exactly are the pregnancy hormones, and which ones do what? After all it's not as if those medical professors sit around in the university and hospital meeting rooms going, "Ooh, you know, pregnancy hormones, whatever they're called." At least I hope not. Many of the pregnancy hormones are produced by the placenta, the organ inside the uterus that sustains the developing baby through the umbilical cord. This is kind of a neat trick as the placenta comes out just after your baby does, right when you won't need those hormones any more.

◎ The "thin blue line" hormone is called human chorionic gonadotrophin (HCG). HCG in pee triggers a "positive" result in pregnancy tests. A high level during the first 3 months is one of the suspected reasons for nausea. HCG stimulates the ovaries to produce more progesterone, which in turn shuts down the monthly period department for the duration of the pregnancy.

◎ The "Oh my God, look at these bazoombas" hormones needed for milk production are human placental lactogen (HPL), prolactin, estrogen, and progesterone. HPL is responsible for enlarging the breasts and the secretion of colostrum, the "premilk" or "practicing milk," which may leak from your nipples from about the fifth month (or not) and is produced for the first few days after the birth.

◎ Relaxin, the "hang loose" pregnancy hormone, makes ligaments and tissues soften up and become more elastic, which provides the increased flexibility in the joints of the pelvis and back needed for labor. It may also contribute to the "waddle" of later pregnancy. (The other contributing factor being that you've turned into a giant wombat.)

◎ Oxytocin is the squeezer hormone: it stimulates contractions of the uterus. Injections of a synthentic version of this hormone, pitocin, are often used to induce labor and to expel the placenta.

⑥ The "coloring-in" hormone is melanocyte-stimulating hormone (MSH). In the later months of pregnancy, high levels of MSH can make your nipples darken and can cause dark patches on your face and a dark vertical line down the middle of your tummy called the linea nigra (Latin for "black line").

⑥ One of the big two girlie hormones, progesterone affects every aspect of pregnancy. It's produced by the ovaries when you're not pregnant, but eventually the placenta takes over the task during pregnancy. It relaxes smooth muscle: in the uterus so it's less likely to contract and cause miscarriage, and in the bladder, intestines, bowel, and veins so they're more flexible as they're squashed by the growing uterus. It increases your body temperature and breathing rate, causes dilated blood vessels, which can reduce blood pressure and make you feel faint and nauseated, and helps produce breast milk. Immediately after the birth, the level drops and continues to drop for a number of days.

⑥ The other major girlie hormone, estrogen (or more correctly a group of estrogens), is also produced by the ovaries and then the placenta during pregnancy. Estrogens help make everything in the reproductive department behave as it should throughout the pregnancy, including the breasts (enlarging nipples and developing milk glands), the uterus (strengthening), and body tissue (softening). Many believe that excess estrogens cause nausea in the first three months. As with progesterone, the relatively high level of estrogen drops immediately after the birth and continues to drop in the days that follow.

⑥ Endorphins, which mimic the effects of morphine and help blunt perceptions of pain and stress, are hormones produced by the brain up until and during childbirth. After the birth the levels drop sharply. This has been implicated in the temporary "baby blues" most new mothers experience, and the more lasting feelings of depression that sometimes follow. One new mother complained, "They've turned off my happy hormones."

your record

What are your fears and hopes for the pregnancy?

WEEK 13

what's going on Your tummy is probably starting to stick out. Soon it will seem to "pop" and everyone will begin noticing. Any nausea will probably stop or trail off about now.

Down in fetusland, reflexes for sucking, swallowing, and breathing have begun. The amniotic sac surrounding the fetus is full of 100 milliliters of amniotic fluid, a fully appointed unit still with lots of room to bob around in. The ears are finished but can't hear yet. The lungs, liver, kidneys, and digestive bits are still maturing. The head has been growing more slowly than the body since week 11. By the end of this week almost everything should be formed and ready to grow. But the fetus almost certainly wouldn't survive on its own because the organs wouldn't function well enough. Weight: about 1 ounce.

Diary

I am so grumpy. All I want is an extensive personal staff to clean the house, fluff the pillows, cook my dinner, and suck up to me. I have injured myself by sneezing in the middle of a yoga stretch. It felt like I tore through muscles or ligaments on each side of my tummy, down low near the hip bones. Damn exercise: it's bad for you.

And there is far too much drivel written these days about balanced meals for the pregnant woman. A perfectly nutritious and attractive meal can be had by eating three pieces of peanut butter toast and half a carton of chocolate milk in seven seconds flat. Although it is true that I'd probably be dead if I wasn't taking all those vitamins (but not vitamin A, which you can't take if you're preggers).

It's the weirdest thing being nauseous and getting no fun out of food, but still feeding your face relentlessly.

My gums keep bleeding. This is obviously some sort of design fault. Again, many of the books are hopeless, presuming the "mother-to-be" has the brain of the average anteater: "The baby hormones may be making your gums bleed. Take special care with dental hygiene." I always lose consciousness at about the word "hygiene." Beck suggests more vitamin C and that seems to help. Maybe I just had scurvy.

weepiness

At times during pregnancy you can feel ecstatic, elated, like a fertile winged mythical love goddess (well, okay, maybe not), contented, confident, optimistic, and relaxed. But you can also feel depressed, terrified, worried, tense, crabby, moody, and like a blundering water buffalo. Tears are almost inevitable.

Sometimes it can seem that you're on a hair-trigger. Anything can suddenly set you off: sad movies or news stories about bad things that happen to babies or mothers. The rest of the world goes on despite your pregnancy, and with a bit of bad luck yours might coincide with a relationship breakup, other personal complications, or a death in the family.

Even without extra stress, you can feel miserable, especially during the first trimester when your hormones seem to be stuck on the spin cycle. Maybe you recognize some of the symptoms from PMS (premenstrual syndrome). About 10 percent of women have mild to moderate depression while pregnant.

Your moodiness might be manifested by you being cranky and overcritical, or flying into rage or panic about something that isn't really so important, or crying for no specific reason. Or at the long-distance phone ads.

Thinking about pregnancy and becoming a parent can bring up unresolved issues you may have with your own mother and father, or feelings of sadness or anger about your own childhood. And it's natural to feel ambivalent about being pregnant, and worried about many aspects of pregnancy and parenting, and grieving for a lifestyle lost.

Your pregnancy worries can include (but are not strictly limited to) the following.

Will my baby be born healthy and "normal"? (Very probably.)

Do I deserve a healthy baby? (Oooh, yes.)

How will I juggle parenting and career? (You won't know until you get there, but you can talk to people who do it and see if any of their strategies might suit you.)

How will I cope with childbirth? (The best way you can.)

Sleep deprivation? (Get all the sleep you can now.)

Breastfeeding? (There's lots of help available, and in the end it isn't compulsory.)

Curtailed freedom? (There are compensations. But yes. Life ain't perfect.)

And loss of autonomy? (It will pass in about 20 years or so.)

Will I have "maternal instincts"? (Being a good parent is about being kind, patient, and ready to learn, not about "instincts.")

Will I bond with my baby? (Probably, and if you don't there is lots of help available.)

How will my relationship with my partner be affected? (You'll probably both be sleep-deprived and grumpy for a while. Express your fears and keep talking.)

How will my partner cope with the demands of parenting? (Don't know, but there's lots of help available.)

Will my baby suffer from me being a single parent? (Children need a stable, loving environment. You can do that.)

Will I ever recognize my body again? (Yes, and you should stop looking at photos of famous actresses and models who have had children. They also have forty-seven nannies, personal trainers, and teeming hordes of hair and makeup artists.)

How will I/we cope with a reduced income and increasing expenses? (Have a strategy.)

Why wouldn't you have the occasional wave of panic when you remember any or all of the above, plus the fact that your life is about to be transformed, and there's no going back?

Maybe you just need a good cry every now and then or to share your feelings with your partner or a friend. If a particular issue is really getting you down, or if you feel depressed most of the time, it might help to get some professional counseling. It's better to sort things out now than when you have a real, live, nontheoretical baby on your hands: talk to your doctor.

Here's the bit everyone bangs on about, but only because it's true: if you're feeling really upset, don't guzzle alcohol and caffeine and stuff your face with junk food. Eat a healthy diet, and get yourself some exercise, fresh air, and plenty of rest.

Partners and friends, who are always on the lookout for a way to help you, should be ordered to cheer you up. And you need to hang out with some cheerful parents.

the way people react to the news

When people react to your pregnancy, it's not about you, it's about them. If they say negative or rude things, it comes from their own experience or their own personality, their own fears, or their own problems with body image, babies, their mother, whatever. Every time you hear something discouraging ("Your life is over") or ludicrous ("Childbirth doesn't hurt at all"), just say to yourself, "It's not about me, it's about them."

what's going on

The second trimester kicks off this week. You'll probably start to feel a bit more energetic. With a bit of luck the nausea should be gone or almost gone. You may get a dark line from your navel to the top of your bikini line. This is called the linea nigra because doctors think "black line" sounds soooo much more sophisticated in Latin. On white skin it's not a black line: it varies from a pale, shadowy pink to a browny color. On dark skin it can look darker, or not be visible at all. You will almost certainly be "showing"—have a bump in your tummy. According to the fruit-metaphor brigade your uterus is the size of a large grapefruit.

By now an expert ultrasound operator can often see whether the fetus is a boy or a girl, by the presence or absence of a suspiciously willylike object. The bones are forming in the arms, legs, rib cage, and skull. It's the start of your baby's skeleton. Weight: about 1 1/2 ounces.

DiARy I've stopped being grumpy and started being weepy. I'm trying to regard this as progress. I'm getting more forgetful: this might be pregnancy hormones, or just having more to think about. So much for the alleged energy surge of the second trimester that everyone goes on about . . . I feel a little better by the end of the week. At least the nausea's gone and only pays a surprise visit now and again.

I investigate my sneezing/yoga injury. There is a muscle called the psoas that extends from the lower back to the front groin and I have injured mine waving my legs in the air. My chiropractor, the second-most sensible woman in the world (strangely not called Lorraine), gives me an extremely gentle exercise to do three times a day and says a walk of 10 minutes or so at a time is plenty until it gets better. She can't feel around because the fetus is in the way, and she says since everything is changing in the pelvis, healing the muscle isn't going to be top priority for my body.

I decide that my ill-fated attempts at yoga are simply a joke. If you're not already a yoga enthusiast you can end up injuring yourself. On the other hand, if you are the sort of person who ties herself up into a pretzel every Wednesday night, if you stretch every day and can climb up your own left leg, well, there's no problem. I should have taken instruction from an exercise person who is trained in pregnancy—I suspect that a lot of people who work in gyms or conduct yoga classes say they know about pregnancy exercise but don't really.

Beck asks whether I've had any puffiness. Nobody mentioned puffiness. There had better not be any puffiness. I'm against it. I've got enough to deal with, thank you very much.

The fact that I feel like I weigh about 56,795 pounds is beginning to depress me. Beck says I will have to exercise from week 20 on, but I shouldn't do too much exercise before then because my system would be not so much shocked as horrified.

"But what about the people who swim 3 miles a day and hike around Montana when they're pregnant?" I ask.

"They are not your type," she replies.

She's right.

I buy a bunch of pregnancy magazines at the newsstand, call in sick, and plop on the couch. Some of them seem pretty reliant on freebies. I remind myself that a whizzbang product being given away is probably not in the magazine because it's necessarily the best or safest thing. It's there because its manufacturers get a free plug and a picture of their stuff in the mag.

One magazine actually gives away baby walkers even though an article in the same issue says they are not recommended for kids because they can slow real walking progress and cause spinal and neck problems.

Another one, called *Fit Pregnancy* is very focused on image, "training" (exercise), and diet, with pages of suggested menus. All those models in the pictures seem to go through pregnancy a size 6 with a cantaloupe up their micro-mini dress. How appalling of me not to look like a whippet in a wig and cook up some Tuscan, three-course, delicious, low-fat, gourmet meal every 2 minutes.

One mag claims to have "Amazing facts about pregnancy and birth." And they're right. They *are* amazing. "A child born feet first will have the power of healing later in life." This is such amazing crap it makes you doubt some of the rest, such as "The heaviest baby born to a healthy mother weighed more than 22 pounds."

info

second-trimester hassles

This is often the most comfortable trimester of the pregnancy. For most women, nausea stops or decreases, energy levels are up, and mood swings moderate. However, in this trimester, you may need to deal with one or more of the following.

sore, bleeding gums

Your gums may develop gingivitis, becoming sore, puffy, inflamed, and prone to bleeding, especially when you brush your teeth. This is caused by the increased progesterone and estrogen in your blood, which makes gums softer and increases the blood pressure in the capillaries at the point where gums and teeth meet. This makes gums more susceptible to damage from food and being bumped by your toothbrush.

Try daily flossing, frequent brushing with a soft toothbrush (after each snack or meal if possible), and at least one dental visit during pregnancy for a professional cleaning job. (Make sure the dentist knows you're pregnant so you're not given an X-ray or medication. Many dentists say local anesthetics are safe during pregnancy.)

Proper levels of calcium, vitamin C, and other nutrients will also help. As well, avoid eating toffeelike stuff or sticky date puddingy things that can get stuck in all the nooks and crannies and encourage infection.

congested nose

Something else you may share with the pregnancy sisterhood is a blocked, congested nose or one that is runnier than usual. You may also get nosebleeds. These schnoz problems are the result of the same hormonal effect that creates gum problems, which causes an increased blood supply, softening and swelling of the mucous membranes inside the nostrils, increased mucus production, and easier bleeding. This means colds and upper respiratory tract infections can take longer than usual to clear up.

Bleeding can be triggered by unrestrained honking (overstrenuous nose blowing) or even by a dry atmosphere, which can harden mucus and make it more likely to cause damage to mucous membranes when you blow your nose. Try to avoid allergens. Humidifying the atmosphere and making yourself steam inhalations can help relieve the symptoms. You can also rub some emollient cream inside each nostril at bedtime.

To stop your nose bleeding apply gentle pressure on the affected side of the nose while leaning your head forward. Frequent or heavy nose bleeding should be mentioned to your doctor. Don't use any nose drops or sprays without checking first with your doctor. And . . . er . . . hate to sound like your granny, but don't pick your nose.

vaginal secretions

I realize this is hardly dinner party conversation, but you'll be pleased to know that all those extra-wet panties are actually normal. Your vagina is producing more mucus and I think it's time we had a better term. Like lady's lotion. God. Sorry. Maybe not.

It's caused by the combined effect again of progesterone and estrogen: the softer, more swollen mucous membranes of pregnancy produce more secretions. (Unpoetically, the medical description is "an increase of normal mucoid discharge," which sounds like something a special-effects technician would say on the set of a critter movie.)

This normal discharge, called leukorrhea if you want to get technical, should be clear or milky white. There can be rather a lot of it, and it's likely to increase as the pregnancy progresses.

To help with the hassle of vaginal secretions in overdrive:

⊚ avoid tight undies or pants.

⊚ wear undies and pants made from natural fabrics such as cotton or wool—avoid nylon and polyester.

⊚ wear panty liners and change them frequently during the day.

⊚ don't use tampons when you're pregnant because there is a higher risk of vaginal infection.

@ if it's easy, take a couple of changes of underpants with you in your handbag (and if you think you need a bigger handbag to leave the house now, just wait until you have a baby!).

Increased blood flow to the genitals can mean a more sensitive than usual clitoris (another reason to stay away from tight undies or pants). (Or not.)

infections

If your vaginal discharge is yellowish or greenish or has an unhealthy smell, you have probably got an infection, which will need to be treated. An imbalance of friendly and unfriendly bacteria and high estrogen levels in the vagina can make you more prone than usual to yeast infections, also known as candida, which may need to be treated by a doctor who knows you're pregnant. Symptoms include a curdlike white discharge and an itching and burning feeling.

If you are having yeast infections, remember to be careful to wipe from front to back after going to the bathroom. This is because yeast can hang out in the bowel and be transferred to your vagina. Yeast infection is linked to a high sugar and yeast diet, so try avoiding refined sugars, and eat lots of yogurt with live *Lactobacillus acidophilus* cultures.

Air the nether regions when possible. You may do this by running around in the nude and waving your legs in the air, or by doing things like wearing no clothes or a nightie to bed instead of pajamas. If you're lucky enough to have warm weather, wear a sarong or skirt with no undies when you can, and avoid staying in a wet swimsuit for hours.

your record

How are you feeling now that you're in the
second trimester? Check the applicable boxes.

❏ better

❏ happy as a clam

❏ get out of my way, I'm going to throw up

❏ excited about my changing body

❏ like my wardrobe just shrank to one ensemble and
a queen-size sleeping-bag

❏ full of beans

❏ completely exhausted, now that you mention it

1

2

3

4

5

6

7

8

what's going on
Your heart is doing a lot more than it used to and has a lot more blood to pump. (Contrary to old ludicrous persons' tales, your heart doesn't actually get bigger.) Nausea might come back if you let yourself get too tired or hungry. You may be looking even more divine than usual as your hair isn't falling out at the rate it normally does, so it looks thicker, your skin looks plumped out, and the extra blood in your system is giving you what they call the glow.

The fetal fingernails are developing, and the facial features are clearly defined. The fetus may suck its thumb. (All together now: awwwwww!) The skin formed is still very thin, so if there were a tiny camera in there transmitting pictures you could see blood vessels underneath. The fetus begins to put on weight more rapidly about this time. Starting soon the arms and legs will begin to be more coordinated when moving—imagine languid fetal aerobics.

Weight: about 3 ounces.

DiARY Matt and I go for a tour of the maternity ward at the hospital we're booked into. Our tour of Maternity is conducted by a very capable, nurse-type Lorraine. In the nursery we look at babies in plastic boxes with the tops cut off. I mean, they're posh plastic boxes on wheels, not homemade or anything.

Because they are in the middle of being renovated, the delivery suites and private rooms look like tacky country motel rooms after being trashed by a desultory heavy metal band. Awful, hideous, floral, flouncy bedspreads I couldn't possibly give birth on. Afterwards I remonstrate with my obstetrician.

"They like things to be feminine," he says.

"Herb," I point out, "if you're squatting down with a baby coming out of your vagina, I reckon you'd know you're a woman."

Some random realities: Sunday. Valentine's Day. We realize we've forgotten our anniversary nearly a month before. Start eating Cheerios all the time. Drag myself around. Leg hurting. The bottom half of me is a milk-white sea of cellulite.

I'm starting to have the feeling that there's no going back. Getting to bed far too late, then not sleeping, then waking early and being unable to get back to sleep, then finally sleeping in and being late for work. I think I may have jet lag, without any jetting.

Nausea gone except when I allow myself to get tired and hungry. Peeing all night long. The idea of wearing my normal clothes—e.g., anything with a ZIPPER or WAIST—is totally laughable. And the books say, "You won't be showing yet." Showing? I'm not just showing! I'm showing OFF!

Searching for maternity clothes in the shops is like wading through the rejects of every other season. A few years ago it was orange and lime-green clothes for women—so now it must be orange and lime-green maternity wear. Cack!

As a clothes designer I know people try to reduce costs by cutting things thinner rather than wider, and shorter rather than longer, but in this case it seems pretty damn stingy. You don't want to be in a hobble skirt when you're already going to be waddling, surely? And why is there nothing between mini- and maxi-length? It's as if only Queen Victoria and one of Rod Stewart's girlfriends buy maternity clothes.

I end up buying sensible items in black—two pairs of pants, one T-shirt, one sweater, a dress, two pairs of tights—and hand over the equivalent of Turkey's national debt. You'd think they had emeralds sewn into the hems. And that's in the normal maternity shop. The posh maternity shop has shiny polyester jackets that aren't meant to be shiny for $250 and various other rich-lady outfits. I look like the *Titanic* in all of them.

info

exercise exercise exercise

Moderate exercise during pregnancy is good for you and your off-spring. When we say moderate exercise, we do not mean flinging yourself about like a nonpregnant person with a gym obsession and a desire to go run a marathon before lunch. Sensible exercise is good for circulation, relaxation, and energy levels and helps to stop constipation, cramps, and backache.

If you're not fit before pregnancy, this is not the time to adopt a strenuous exercise regime. Try things like walking, gentle yoga and stretching, swimming, dancing, prenatal exercise classes, and aquarobics. Look for gyms, swimming, and recreation centers or physical therapy clinics that run exercise classes designed for pregnancy and have instructors with a special qualification in pregnancy exercise; at the very least make sure your instructor knows you're pregnant. Check with your obstetrician or prenatal clinic that the exercise you're doing or about to do is safe for you.

Many instructors are not aware of the special risks and strengths of pregnancy. The extra release of the hormone relaxin, which makes your ligaments and joints more stretchy, can make you more prone to injury. Sit-ups are generally a bad idea during pregnancy because they can cause a separation of muscles in your stomach, creating a hernialike effect.

Yoga can help you become aware of how comfortably you are standing, sitting, or lying down. Its breathing and meditation practices can relax you during pregnancy and labor. Special prenatal yoga classes can help with many of the discomforts of pregnancy, as well as improving the body's suppleness and strength for labor. The mind-body-spirit approach of yoga can be a good match for the mind-body-spirit-altering experience of being pregnant.

Even if you've been superfit before pregnancy, you'll need to apply some limitations to your regime. Consult your gym or fitness professional as soon as you know you're pregnant to get some expert advice on exercise modifications, and choose a slower-pace, lighter-impact class and lighter weights.

If you have played sports regularly before pregnancy, you can usually continue until the third trimester, unless it's a sport that can cause impact injuries, such as soccer (contesting for the ball), trick rollerblading (falls), baseball (sliding collisions), water polo (being kicked, accidentally or otherwise), and tennis (rabid opponents prone to attacking you with a racket).

Other activities not recommended during pregnancy include horseback riding, any kind of skiing, scuba diving, backpacking, and lifting heavy weights and other heavy manual work. Jogging, running, and other athletics may be stressful on joints, breasts, and baby, so check your exercise program with your doctor.

You shouldn't exercise while pregnant if you have a history of medical conditions such as recurrent miscarriages, incompetent cervix, preterm birth, or heart disease. Other conditions, including diabetes, thyroid disease, placenta previa, preeclampsia, and anemia, may sometimes mean exercise is not recommended.

when exercising

◎ Wear supportive footwear and a sports bra.

◎ Drink plenty of water before, during, and after, and make sure you have some healthy snacks handy.

◎ Remember your center of gravity is changing, which will affect your balance and coordination, so take it easy.

◎ Listen to and trust your body—stop if any activity makes you feel uncomfortable, overtired, hot, dizzy, faint, or crampy.

◎ Don't worry if your resting heart rate is higher during pregnancy even when you're not exercising. It doesn't mean you are losing fitness; it simply reflects your increased rate of circulation.

◎ Don't get overheated for prolonged periods—this can be damaging to the fetus, particularly during the first trimester.

◎ Exercise intensity should be measured during workouts; a fetal heart rate stays normal when exercise intensity is moderate and your heart rate doesn't exceed 140 beats per minute (bpm), whereas if your heart rate reaches 180 bpm this can cause fetal distress and a lowered fetal heart rate. You can wear one of those pulse monitor thingies (that's the technical term) to check your heart rate.

◎ You can walk until you are slightly puffing or reach 140 bpm, then keep this up for 15–20 minutes. Puffing workouts should be done only every second day and depend on your fitness level.

◎ Go gently with abdominal exercises, and support your tummy with your interlinked hands while doing them; about 30 percent of women have a separation of the abdominal muscles. If this happens, you need to stop any exercising that affects the area.

◎ Strictly limit exercises that involve lying flat on your back to a maximum of 2–3 minutes, especially from the beginning of the second trimester, and omit them altogether after you reach 20 weeks. The weight of the uterus can compress the inferior cava vena, the vein that carries blood back to your heart from your lower parts, ultimately resulting in a reduced blood flow to your head and to the baby. So if you feel dizzy or faint while on your back, turn onto your left side and rest.

◎ Don't forget to exercise your pelvic-floor muscles (Kegel exercises)—these muscles are like a hammock or sling that sits underneath all your inside organs and has holes in it corresponding to the various openings to the outside. Tighten your pelvic-floor muscles, as though you are trying to stop a pee, three or four times a day. Do as many of these as you can before getting tired. Every prenatal exercise class will tell you how important these are. Doing the exercises will mean faster pelvic-floor recovery after delivery, and will help prevent accidental peeing (also known as stress incontinence) when you sneeze, cough, or laugh after childbirth.

 See also Exercise in Help.

your record

What exercise did you do before pregnancy?

What exercise are you doing now?

1

2

3

4

5

6

7

8

what's going on

It is possible you might feel the movements of the fetus as "butterflies" in your stomach from now on, especially if you know what to pay attention to, but you also might not feel it for weeks.

You now have about 180 milliliters of amniotic fluid. Your uterus is kind of like a balloon full of yellowish water. All the joints of the fetus are working and the fingers and toes are all there and waving about. Toenails are just starting to form. The head still looks kind of oversized but the rest of the body is catching up. The downy fetal hair called lanugo has started to grow on the body. (Lanugo means fine wool in some ancient language.) There are various opinions about what the lanugo might be for: it might help keep the fetus warm, or it might be an underfelt for the gooey stuff that eventually covers the baby. Or maybe the fetus is just trying to develop a fashion instinct.

Weight: about 4 ounces.

WIN!

VATS OF

VOGUE

DiARY
No idea what happened this week.
Blinked and missed it.
Oprah's hair's looking magnificent though,
I must say.

Reading for Dads·to·Be

info

'fess up to being pregnant

You're slower, you're more tired, you're more spacey, especially in the first 3 months, and apparently we've got it to look forward to again in the last 3 months. (That leaves these middle 3 months in which everyone tells us we're looking divine, just glowin' up a storm.) Tell people you're tired. Let them help. And let them make allowances. Forgot to pay the phone bill? It's because you're pregnant. Have to sit down on the floor during a meeting and put your feet on a chair and show everyone your undies? Because you're pregnant. Had to buy a new pair of red shoes? Pregnant. See? It's easy.

the pursed-lip brigade

Not married? Married but wearing tight clothes? Planning to go back to work before the baby turns 17? Somewhere, somehow, someone will disapprove of you. Get used to it. If you stay home with the baby, some idiots will start asking, "What do you DO all day?" as if you're just sitting at home watching *Oprah* and eating Mars Bars (ahem). If you're at work, people will ask, "You haven't put your baby in child care/hired a nanny, have you?" as if it were the same as asking, "You haven't tied your baby to a tree for a day, have you?" Apply the same logic as you do for unsolicited advice: it's not about you, it's about them.

stuff you didn't know before

1. Breast milk comes out of the nipple like water comes out of a sprinkler—there are heaps of little holes, not just one. And one breast may produce heaps more milk than the other.

2. What the inside of your navel looks like.

3. You *can* want to throw up and eat at the same time.

4. You *can* go and pee all the time and still retain fluid.

5. Sleep deprivation starts well before the birth.

stuff that people don't know

It makes people be nicer to you when they know:

⑥ you are carrying a quarter more blood than you usually do.

⑥ in the second half of the pregnancy the baby whacks you in the internal organs all the time, and it's not always a cute little whack— sometimes it's really uncomfortable, sometimes it actually hurts.

⊚ your feet swell to twice their usual size (well, that's what it feels like).

⊚ you can't get the required amount of deep sleep because you have to pee all night—it's the equivalent of someone waking you up every couple of hours.

stuff for guys

Warning: We're assuming your partner is a man for the next few paragraphs.

If your partner won't read or learn anything about childbirth, at least tell him:

a) there's going to be a lot of blood.

b) there's not much he can do about the pain, and that's not his job.

c) the obstetrician or midwife may well feel the medical necessity to put their hand all the way inside you—this is not a cue for your partner to say, "Watch out!"

d) if he thinks he is going to faint, he should put his head between his knees or stand on tippytoes, or go outside and have a rest. (I say let's see 'im try all three at once.)

BOOKS AND SITES FOR GUYS

Most of the books available for men aren't much use as "how to" manuals for dads who are at home being the "primary caregiver," but guys can read the usual books and stuff that's aimed at moms (see Baby-Care Books in Week 43). After all, it's the same problems and the same advice. Except if you count the stuff about boobs.

So You're Going to Be a Dad by Peter Downey, Perseus Publishing, Cambridge, MA, 2002.

Hilarious book from the engagingly honest Mr. Downey: one to make fathers-to-be laugh out loud. There are quite a few practical hints for dads, mostly working ones rather than stay-at-home ones, and lots of stories that see the funny side of stuff like . . . well, poop.

Babyhood by Paul Reiser, Avon, New York, 1997.
Comedian and star of *Mad About You* Paul Reiser gives a stand-up-style account of becoming a dad.

Keeping the Baby Alive till Your Wife Gets Home by Walter Roark, Clearing Skies Press, Atlanta, GA, 2001.
A funny look at being a dad.

Fathermag.com
A magazine on the Web for dads.

The Joy of Fatherhood: The First Twelve Months by Marcus Jacob Goldman, M.D., Crown Publishing Group, New York, 2000.
Lots of help with how to adjust to your new life—and keep stuff in it you already liked, such as friends. Includes practical stuff such as how to tell if baby is sick.

The New Father: A Dad's Guide to the First Year AND **The New Father: A Dad's Guide to the Toddler Years** by Armin Brott, Abbeville Press, New York, 1997.
A boxed set featuring advice from "experts" and real dads on all sorts of subjects including child development, changing relationships, and men's feelings.

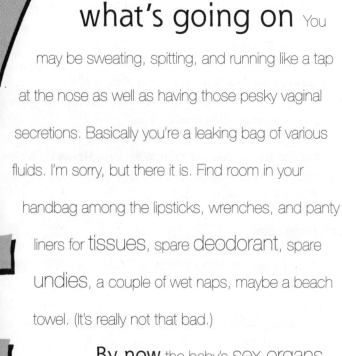

what's going on You

may be sweating, spitting, and running like a tap

at the nose as well as having those pesky vaginal

secretions. Basically you're a leaking bag of various

fluids. I'm sorry, but there it is. Find room in your

handbag among the lipsticks, wrenches, and panty

liners for tissues, spare deodorant, spare

undies, a couple of wet naps, maybe a beach

towel. (It's really not that bad.)

By now the baby's sex organs

are completely formed. The fetal kidneys

produce lots of urine: the fetus pees about

every 40–45 minutes (at least you don't have to

change diapers yet). Icky though it may

sound, the fetus takes in some of this pee

when it swallows mouthfuls of

amniotic fluid. But most of the fetal

waste products go through the placental

membrane and into your circulation, where they are

dealt with by your body's usual functions.

Weight: about 5¼ ounces.

STARTLING
BOSOMS

Diary — My boobs are getting bigger, and none of my bras are comfy, even the bigger ones I bought. My bosoms used to stick out straight from my body, practically in opposite directions from each other. They were known as East and West. Now they're kind of bigger and lower slung, meaning there's a bit underneath where it gets sweaty. And all these little skin tags have grown there as well. Thank God I finally found a book that said this was perfectly normal.

Sport tank tops seemed the best, but now they feel like elastic-bandage boob-tubes three sizes too small. If I'm sitting around at home I don't wear a bra at all. No doubt this means I'll end up having boobs shaped like tube socks that I can tie in a knot behind my neck when they get in the way. Don't care. Those areas around my nipples I can never pronounce have started to go brown and are getting bumps on them.

Farewell, my strawberries-and-cream nipples, my horizontal, pointy bosoms! Will you now both be called South forever? Why don't I have a photo of you?! Was my youth so misspent that I never even posed for nude photographs? What was I thinking!

I'm feeling very annoyed with myself for not being a supple, lithe, yoga-frenzied woman.

The bathtub in the new house is of such a ludicrous design by some kind of deranged handyman that before I can get in it I have to crawl over about half a yard of tiles or take a huge, dangerous step on one leg. (Well, obviously, otherwise it would be a jump, not a step. I'm losing my mind.) And given that there isn't enough room in the bathroom to swing a cat—actually there isn't even enough room to *shout* at a cat—it won't do. The whole thing is a disaster waiting to happen for a woman whose center of gravity is changing every day.

I call Bud the plumber to come and fix it. (All sensible handyman types are called Bud, just as all sensible women are called Lorraine.) Bud, of course, finds that the bathroom floor is practically rotted through as well and that there's some other piping-style disaster, which means the job turns out to be five times bigger.

One of the reasons I feel like I'm going mad is sleep deprivation. It never occurred to me this would happen BEFORE the little tyke arrived. One of the books says this is because I'm sleeping like a baby—not much deep sleep but plenty of REM sleep. That stands for Rapidly Enraged Mother-to-be.

Call me dense, but it's only just hit me I'm not one person who's pregnant—I mean, I am—but I'm also two people. No. I'm not two people but there are two people—a big one and a little one—sharing the same body. Well. That's a bit spooky.

Matt's reading bits of a book for wannabe fathers, which argues that men shouldn't be expected to be at the birth because they can't fix the pain, and if they prefer, they can plant a tree or invent a new dance instead, to celebrate the birth. I'm afraid Matt is the sort of guy who thinks this is a load of crap, and the way that book is being hurled about it won't last the evening. I don't think he's the making-up-a-dance type.

info

breasts

Ah, boobs. On the one hand there are the people who go "Phwoaaarrr" and, on the other, people who worship them as sacred life-giving vessels of compulsorily acquired nourishment. Get a grip. They're just boobs.

Probably one of the first pregnancy changes you noticed were your breasts getting larger and more tender. They'll keep growing, but extreme sensitivity usually settles down after the first trimester. From here on, the hormones estrogen, progesterone, and prolactin stimulate more growth and the production of some premilk stuff called colostrum.

Each breast contains about twenty segments or lobes; each of these is made up of grapelike bunches of glands called alveoli; and each of these is lined with milk-producing cells. During pregnancy your bosoms get bigger because not only do your dormant milk-producing cells and ducts enlarge but your body also grows new ones to help out. (Your original breast size bears no relation to milk production.)

the changes

Breast changes are usually more extreme in a first pregnancy. Your breasts may feel tender, tingling, warm, full, heavy, painfully sensitive, or lumpy. You may even have some stabbing pain.

You'll be able to see more veins, often blue, close to the skin's surface, carrying the extra blood supply to the area. They're especially noticeable if you have fair skin.

The nipples and areolae (the areas around each nipple) become larger and darker, particularly if your natural skin tone is dark. Most nipples and areolae go a shade of brown, even if they have been pink before. This can happen gradually to the entire area, or in patches.

Each areola is dotted with sebaceous (oil-producing) glands called Montgomery's tubercles (those little bumps), which secrete a fluid that keeps the nipples supple. The glands become more prominent during pregnancy, so you get a bumpier effect.

You may have a small amount of colostrum—a thin, yellowish liquid—leaking from your nipples toward the end of pregnancy, and even earlier on, but not everyone does. This can cause wet patches but can be soaked up and hidden by breast pads, otherwise known as nursing pads; you can buy these in the baby section of the drugstore or supermarket. Actual milk production won't start until after the baby arrives.

bras

Wearing a well-fitted supporting bra during pregnancy is recommended. You often need to increase your bra measurement and cup size by at least one size. The increase might even be more, depending on the overall weight gain and whatever your breasts feel like doing. (For example, you might go from 34B to 36C.) You can buy bras to fit your changing size, even though it might mean buying a new size a couple of times during the pregnancy. You don't need a nursing bra (with front fasteners that make for easy bosom access) or new size while your present bra fits well, is comfortable, and gives you enough support.

Good features of a nursing bra include wide straps, a wide band of fabric under the breast, and a high cotton content. Anything that digs into the skin is even more intolerable than usual, so make sure you get a comfy fit.

Nursing bras often fasten at the front between the cups; or where the straps meet the cups at the front; or they don't fasten at all, but rather stretch down so you can just pop a boob out the top to breastfeed. Whatever suits you best. If you started with big bosoms, you'll probably need more support than the stretchy tank-top style.

afterward

Don't be sucked in by cosmetic surgery hype that breasts are "deformed" by breastfeeding and need to be "enlarged" with sacs of plastic and saline. Sharky cosmetic surgeons don't really care about your bosoms, they just want your money. And there are many possible hideous side effects, including rupture, pain, scarring, lost nipple sensation, and inability to breastfeed again.

Likewise beware the quacky marketing techniques of the cosmetics companies trying to sell you "bust firming" and "breast cream," and "body treatment" moisturizers. (Often the names are in French or pseudo-French.) They will not prevent your breasts from changing shape or sagging. These creams don't affect the tissues inside the breast, and many are a shockingly expensive waste of time. A cheap moisturizer that smells nice is just as good at keeping the surface of your skin moist, and just as likely to keep your breasts firm—that is, not at all.

Often these creams and oils have ingredients that feel tingly or make the skin seem tighter—the same tightening feeling can be achieved by putting egg white on your breasts and waiting for it to dry. Don't be fooled—there's no lasting effect on your bosomry and certainly these creams are no match for Mrs. Gravity once she's decided to make her presence felt.

your record

Do a little drawing of what your breasts used to be like, and what they look like now. Oh, what the hell, draw your whole body or paste in a photo.

what's going on

You'll find many pregnancy books tell you that this is the week you'll start to feel a first baby move around. Don't hold your breath: you might not feel it move for weeks yet, and that doesn't mean there's anything wrong. You mostly notice your baby move when you're resting at night. Use pillows to support your growing tummy while you sleep.

According to some pregnancy experts, this week the fetus can make facial expressions. Oh yeah? Like what? Astonishment? "Euwww yuk, that amniotic fluid tastes bad"? Anyway, the fetus is definitely able to move around a lot, swing on the umbilical cord (well, that's what it looks like), and bite its own fingers or do the hokey-pokey if it feels like it. There is lanugo hair all over the body, and blood cells start to form in the bone marrow. Tastebuds are forming. Weight: about 7 ounces.

DiARY I head off to a group fitness class at the hospital. It is mostly couples, except me, and exactly the sort of thing I hate—name tags and a white board and splitting into two groups to workshop questions such as "What does fitness mean to you?" and "Will exercise help?" (Duh, I think. 'Course it will.)

I am very annoyed to discover that mad exercising in the last few weeks of pregnancy will not actually guarantee a short labor. This seems to be another major design fault of this whole caper, along with painful childbirth.

A woman called Anthea, wearing a black velvet headband on her long blonde hair and shoes that cost more than all the rest of the clothes in the room added together, tells the class smugly that she is still going to gym every day and doing a special program of exercises and weights. She looks really shocking—has a gray pallor and is scarily thin for someone who is pregnant. Lorraine the gym instructor asks her if her personal trainer is qualified to work with pregnant women. No, Anthea says, rather patronizingly, explaining that it's a very superior sort of gym and they do know she's pregnant and IT'S REEEEAL EXPENSIVE.

Later in the class when Lorraine explains a separation of the abdominal muscle that causes bits of your organs to poke through in a line under the skin of your tummy in a characteristic shape, Anthea squeals in recognition, "Oh my GOD, I've got that!" and goes a bit quiet for the rest of the class. One imagines the very superior gym is about to receive a call from her reeeal expensive lawyer.

We practice (a) sitting on giant inflatable balls to strengthen our squatting muscles and straighten our backs, (b) sprawling in beanbags, and (c) a relaxation technique that I fail at miserably. Not for me relaxing, in a hospital room full of strangers lying on nylon carpet with the fluorescent lights temporarily off, thank you. We are informed about the importance of pelvic-floor exercises and I just know I'm not going to do them. I've tried. I did six in a row one Saturday and got bored. We all pass around a plastic pelvis and stare at it as if it might suddenly have something to tell us.

Here's what I learn in the class.

✳ The average female pelvis is ludicrously small for what's expected of it.

✳ Pelvic-floor exercises exercise the pelvic floor (hello). (The pelvic floor is the trampoliney bit that is stretched under all the pelvic organs.) The main jobs of the pelvic floor are to stop all your organs from falling out of your vagina (well, they wouldn't really, but it would all get a bit saggy in there); contracting around the holes to prevent unscheduled leaking, especially during coughing or sneezing (that is, it's a continence accessory); and allowing your vagina to contract rhythmically if you are in any way interested in sex, which is hard to imagine.

✳ How to exercise the pelvic-floor muscles without anybody noticing. My favorite instruction was "Your buttocks should not be moving." I often think that.

✳ They now say to work your pelvic-floor muscles to fatigue three to four times a day, rather than five times thirty times a day or thirty times five times a day, which was the old-fashioned advice.

✳ It is difficult to have a mid-class snack while the instructor is explaining to a young woman how to poop properly. (Tragically, I walked away, so I'll never know.)

✳ Nap when you can, even for 15 minutes.

✳ Bend and rotate your arms backward like you're doing a chicken dance, when you can. Also put your feet up when you can and, if you can't, flex them back and forth. Both of these will keep your muscles flexible and help your circulation.

✳ Don't hunch over your stomach. Sit backward on a chair, with a pillow between you and the chair back and your legs to each side, or sit on a giant inflatable ball, which you can buy from exercise-supply shops.

✳ If you have to pick something up, use the lunge position (bend at the knee, one leg in front, keeping your back straight). If you vacuum, hold the cord behind your back with one hand, which automatically keeps your back straight. When you're at the sink, stand on one leg and put the other foot on the shelf under the sink, as long as the shelf is low enough for you to feel comfortable. Anthea says what are we thinking of, we should all hire a housekeeper. (I suggest we could dress her in a long, black dress and call her Mrs. Danvers.)

✳ A diagram of a uterus looks like a bagpipe with a tent rope on it.

✳ Being fit may not ensure an easy labor, but it may mean a better labor and recovery than you would have had if you were unfit.

✳ Don't go into hot tubs, Jacuzzis, steam rooms, or saunas. Their temperature can be raised to dangerous levels for the fetus without you realizing it.

✳ Don't get really hot and then jump in a cold pool, or otherwise shock your system with sudden temperature changes.

✳ Because the relaxin hormone goes into overdrive during pregnancy and slackens all the ligaments, joints, and muscles, don't overstretch or bounce on stretches.

Jill, who'll probably be a godmother without the God bit, and Matt come to this week's ultrasound. I'm a bit nervous. In my heart I feel that everything is fine but my head is saying, well, things do go wrong. My left ankle just doesn't know what to think. Actually it probably has nothing to do with my head—instead it's got a microprocessor implanted by Aunt Peg to flash signals at me regularly throughout life: "TERRIBLE things can happen."

It all turns out all right. Going by the pictures on the screen the fetus is 17 weeks 4 days, but ultrasounds only provide "guesstimates." Jill is pretty thunderstruck. I think she was expecting it to be a fairly static side view. Instead the "camera" goes in from all angles—top of head, soles of feet—and measures the length of the thighbone and the arm bone, and thankfully everything's all right and connected to the other right bits.

The fetus face still looks pretty spooky, sort of like a skeleton face with black shapes where the eyes should be. The shot of the spine makes our little darling look like the remains of a flounder on a dinner plate. It's hard not to think it's really waving or having a chat or playing peekaboo when really all it's doing is instinctively having a rowdy time, practicing grabbing, sucking, and tap dancing. Dr. Donaldson takes quite some time and is very thorough, checking the four valves of the heart, measuring a whole lot of circumferences and lengths and widths. He speaks very quietly to his assistant, who types it all into a computer.

Matt and I turn up afterward at Dr. Herb's and I take one look at the waiting room, which looks like an upper-middle-class refugee camp or a headband convention, before rolling my eyes at Lorraine and saying, "I just had a clear ultrasound and I'm going home." She agrees, and accepts a small bottle of my pee as a token of her gratitude.

"Shall I weigh myself or just get out?"

"Just get out," she says. Good old Lorraine.

Suddenly sleeping a lot better and floating through the days. If I didn't know better I'd say I was on drugs.

Another thing I have started noticing: people who warn you against unsolicited advice already have their own. "Don't listen to any busybodies," they say. "What you'll need to do is . . . "

<u>info</u>

repelling unwanted advice and comments

When people give you that firm advice—"You *must* have a nanny," "You *must* always look after the baby yourself," "*Men* can't look after babies," "You *must* use disposable diapers."—remember it's about them, not you. They're usually just telling you what THEY did and insisting that you do the same, maybe partly because that's all they know and partly because if you do it the same way it will make them feel better. Don't forget: your experience will be different from everybody else's. Listen, but don't automatically follow their advice.

It starts as soon as you tell people you're pregnant and continues throughout parenting life. Having babies is such a universal experience that everyone has opinions and advice to share, whether you want to hear them or not.

You'll hear things about whether you can tell if you're having a girl or boy based on how sick you are, how much your baby moves, or what shape your tummy is; why you should only see an obstetrician/midwife; why you should/shouldn't use pain relief drugs during childbirth; how to avoid an episiotomy/cesarean/ cracked nipples; why you must/mustn't breastfeed; why you should always use/never bother with cloth diapers; how you make your baby sleep through the night (pick it up/ignore it/give it a stiff gin); how to avoid diaper rash; why you must go straight back/never go back to work; what sort of child care is best; what sort of schooling is best; what to do when your child is arrested in its mid-thirties. The list seems infinite.

Some advice will be useful and compatible with your own ideas, and some won't. Read books you like the philosophical feel of, and choose a couple of friends to listen to. In the end you'll find that having to deal with your own, real baby will provide the best information.

Another mind-boggling thing is that people want to touch your tummy, and sometimes they don't even ask if it's okay. This is easier to cope with than the advice. You can say, "I'd rather you didn't," or grab hands that are heading toward your belly.

at work or parties

Sometimes people, even in a meeting at work, will bang on about anything to do with pregnancy, including cervical mucus, in front of anyone at all. (Make sure this isn't you.) You can learn to get out of these mortifying situations by saying pleasantly and firmly, "Let's stick to the agenda, shall we?" Even if it's a lie, you can always try, "Oh, I've got a rule—no pregnancy talk at work/parties/whatever," then gently disengage and move away. You can go to the bathroom and come back if you think someone will have changed the subject in the meantime.

strangers

Advice can be worse in your first pregnancy because people assume you want their opinion, and you have no ammunition to defend yourself against it. You can give strangers a distant smile and no verbal response. A lot of pregnancy/baby chitchat when you're out and about is from people who are just looking to pass the time of day or strike up a conversation. These ones are easily dealt with: "Gosh, is that the time? Must fly."

friends

Advice from friends is usually offered with good intentions, and they can give you some invaluable insights and shortcuts. Store away anything that seems useful and ignore anything you don't like the sound of. Alternatively, you can always tell friends you'll come to them if you have any questions, or that you're sick of everybody giving you advice and could they please shut right up before you slap them.

the older generation

Take with a grain of salt any of the pregnancy and baby-care advice from parents or parents-in-law, which is likely to have a long-expired use-by date. It's worth having a tactful chat early on about how you see their role in relation to the baby. Without putting too fine a point on it, they need to understand that as far as the baby goes, you're the boss.

Unfortunately, some members of the older generation, including grandparents, may have fixed ideas about how things should be done (the way they did them). Here are some of the outdated notions you may have to firmly explain are not acceptable.

Before the baby arrives

"Eat lots of lamb and liver." (No, too much vitamin A can damage the fetus.)

"Morning sickness is a myth." (It isn't.)

"You should try to hide your 'bump'." (Oh, for God's sake!)

After the baby arrives

"Breastfeeding/bottle-feeding is bad for your baby." (It's your choice.)

"There's no need to use a baby seat in the car for every trip, particularly short ones." (This is potentially lethal and can lead to horrific injuries.)

"Put the baby to sleep on its tummy." (This is a sudden infant death syndrome—SIDS—risk, according to statistics.)

"Throwing the baby into the air is perfectly okay." (No, this can be as damaging to the brain and eyes as shaking a baby.)

"Put honey on a pacifier." (It rots teeth, can create a "sweet" dependency, and is considered unsafe for a baby less than 12 months old.)

"Spanking, smacking, and threats of violence are good disciplinary measures." (These teach the child to hit other children and creatures smaller than they are.)

"That child is being 'bad.'" (This targets the child, not the behavior.)

"Of course dropping in without calling to check if it's convenient is all right." (Aaaargghhhh!)

"Give small children candy and sugared soft drinks as a treat or a reward. And milk or juice in their nighttime bottles is fine." (All these are a major cause of painful tooth decay.)

"Always leave a baby to cry/never leave a baby to cry even for 30 seconds." (Both of these are extreme.)

"Insist on a sleep routine/refuse to follow a sleep routine." (Whatever works for you is fine.)

Grandparents might say, "But we did this with you and you turned out fine" Rather than replying, "Well, that was darn lucky then, wasn't it?" try saying, in the case of safety issues, "You did the right thing then, but they've done all this new research and the right thing to do now is . . ." When all else fails, just say, "I really need it to be done this way." In the case of safety issues, if a friend or relative is likely to ignore your wishes, it's safer for you to be there whenever they have access to the baby or your older children.

solicited advice

Advice from experts and pregnancy books is often conflicting, which can be confusing. You only need to experience the nurses'-shift changeovers at a hospital when you're learning how to breastfeed to find out just how varied professional opinion can be. It can be tricky to filter it, and—as always—you need to assess the individual you're dealing with, whether it be a physical therapist conducting a prenatal class or a breastfeeding consultant or a pediatrician after the baby's born.

Find women you relate to who are pregnant, or who have had children, especially recently. Ask them anything you need to know, and they'll tell you their experiences. But bear in mind you're just researching—your experiences will not be exactly the same, though you may get pointed in a few directions. New moms will have a few hints about settling babies or the best diapers, that kind of useful stuff. Moms whose kids are older may have forgotten the details.

your record

Write down all the unsolicited and solicited advice you get.

Useful	Not useful

Average approximate fetus length this week from head to butt

1

2

3

4

5

6

7

8

WOMB
SWEET
WOMB

PLENTY of ROOM

WE

what's going on

Your waistline is missing, presumed obliterated. You may have backache, skin pigment changes, and a tendency to vague . . . somethingerother. The fetus still has plenty of room to move around in the amniotic sac, but it's a tighter fit than, say, a pear in a bucket of water—that's why, if you haven't already, you will feel movements any time from now on.

Its muscles have developed enough for the fetus to be doing loop-the-loops. The fetus is putting on fat deposits, which produce heat to keep it warm. Weight: about 9 ounces.

DiARY

I have been reading English pregnancy author Sheila Kitzinger. She abandons comparing the fetus to fruit for a moment to solemnly declare, "You may notice that you are putting on weight on your buttocks." Actually I've been noticing that for the last 19 weeks, Sheila. If they're going to get any bigger, people will start to think I'm shoplifting a futon.

The finance experts in magazines and on the radio all suggest that when you stop using contraception you should start saving for all the stuff you're going to need, especially because one person is probably going to drop an income for a while. Accordingly, we are spending money like it's the last day on earth we can.

I have $105 left in the bank. We've got security screens, we've got built-in closets coming, we've got trees going into the garden. We've got new maternity clothes. For some reason I'm in a frenzy and keep wanting to buy towels even though we've got enough. Must be some innate memory of all those films where the baby's come early and some gnarled old lady shouts, "Boil some towels and splice the mainsail!" Or perhaps I'm thinking of pirate movies. "I've boiled the water and trained the parrot, dear. Everything's going to be fine."

Back, legs, and neck all painful. Get hysterical. Call the chiropractor at home. Make an appointment for the next afternoon, so of course by the next morning after a reasonable sleep (only four or five pees during the night!) most of the symptoms are gone.

Rush from the chiropractor to Dr. Herb's because I skipped seeing him last week after the ultrasound. I can't wait to listen to the heartbeat again. I am beginning to get quite worried because I can't feel the baby move like all the books say I should by now. Maybe Cellsie's gone out.

Thankfully there are no infuriating mothers in the waiting room. Lorraine asks for my pee.

"I gave you some of my pee last week, Lorraine. Now you're just getting greedy."

I sit in the waiting room remembering my weekend of feeling weepy, hideous, fat, disgusting, pimply, and vilely repellent in every degree and getting really freaked out about the sea of cellulite. So far I've been Sneezy, Sleepy, Dopey, and Grumpy. I'm hoping for the full complement of the Seven Dwarfs before the confinement. There wasn't a Weepy, sadly. Or a Crappy. Or a Dippy. Pimply never got a look in. Or, indeed, a Fatty. Can't think why.

Try this out on Dr. Herb, who says I could be Happy. I feel like saying you can be Doc, Doc. When it comes to the crunch I suspect I'm going to be Shrieky, or at least the Evil Queen. Then he tells me somebody has already made the Seven Dwarfs joke in a book he can't remember the name of. Great. So now I'm Plagiary as well.

"Listen, Herb," I say, "all the books say by week 20 you should have felt the baby move, and it's week 19 and mine's gone out for coffee or is playing possum."

Herb's opinion on the matter, basically, is screw the books (except that Dr. Herb probably never says "screw"), I'll feel it soon enough.

I realize that I don't know whether you keep feeling the baby once you've felt it for the first time or if you have to wait another week. Herb says once you feel it you feel it every day. He puts the little instrument on my stomach and it amplifies the baby's heartbeat. It makes me grin.

"It sounds groovy," I say. "Kind of swishy."

"I always think it sounds like new-age massage music," he says. "That wobbly, breathy, deep-sea sound. Anything else worrying you?"

"Yes. I am 171 pounds."

"That's okay."

"Am I putting on too much weight?"

"No, and you can't diet."

"Yes, I know. I was just wondering whether I should rent a wheelbarrow to get around in."

Quite often on the street I suddenly find myself rubbing my stomach in the unselfconscious way men scratch their scrotum. And I don't care who sees me. My stomach sticks way out in front and people ask, "When are you due?" and I say, "August," and they look at me as if I've got a buffalo up my dress. Their next question is usually "Is it twins?"

If it weren't for the phone, I'd never talk to anyone. All my childless friends are busy at work (so am I) and the ones with kids are worse. I never go out at night anymore, and when I do I leave parties at about 10 P.M. stone-cold sober, wishing people wouldn't smoke. Miss Francine was right. My life is over . . .

info

maternity clothes hints

⊚ Length does matter. If you weren't the type to wear a miniskirt before you were pregnant, why would you wear one during pregnancy? Because except for a few ankle-skimmers that's all they make—obviously saving money on materials. In magazines you can even see pregnant models in minidresses wearing long socks, leaving their thighs as the only exposed skin. There are probably only three women in the world who would want to wear this outfit when they're heavily pregnant. If you want a plain dress that ends in the vicinity of your knee, rather than your gusset or your big toe, astonishingly enough, you may have to get someone to make it for you or sew it yourself if you're that way inclined.

⊚ Always remember: this is a TEMPORARY wardrobe. Don't spend a fortune unless you're a diamond heiress, in which case stop reading this book and go and invade Corsica or something.

⊚ Borrow everything you can from a previously pregnant friend, but only things you know you'll wear. Don't clutter up your drawers with stuff that doesn't fit or you wouldn't wear. Write down who has lent you what—with the label and description recorded—so you can give it all back. (Some friends will just say you can pass it on down the line in the great pregnant-women swap meet of life.)

⑥ Don't borrow anything really expensive if the person you're borrowing from wants it back. You never know what could happen to it, and it might be a financial hardship to replace it, even if you could still buy that style, which is unlikely.

⑥ Check out the racks in the following sections: sports, dance wear, men's, and full-figured women's clothes. Bear in mind that in the last month or two of pregnancy just big may not do it. You'll probably need at least a couple of items that have the properly designed stomach bits you only get in maternity clothes.

⑥ Don't worry if your maternity wardrobe is all black, or all navy, or all incredibly boring in some way or other. At least everything will match. You'll be so sick of the sight of your maternity clothes by the time you give birth, anyway, that it doesn't matter.

⑥ Be wary of the pregnancy "kit," which is usually a box containing stretch pants, stretch skirt, a long T-shirt, and a dress. The first company to make the kits was very generous with fabric, but some of the knockoffs and department store copies, while cheaper, are often really stingy with fabric, so everything is tighter and shorter than the original.

⑥ The maternity fashion police will tell you not to wear overalls or stirrup pants because they are unflattering. May I just say that from about the thirty-second week of the pregnancy, you might as well be wearing an armored tank: *nothing* is flattering.

⑥ To cut down on searching every morning, look through your wardrobe ONCE, now. Put all the possible maternity clothes in one spot in your closet and clear a drawer for the non-hanging possible clothes and maternity undies and bras. As each item of normal clothing outlives its usefulness, put it in the normal-person part of the wardrobe or chest of drawers.

⑥ Work out what the weather will be like in the last four months or so of the pregnancy and plan accordingly.

winter

See if any of your friends have a swing coat (also known as an A-line or knee-length overcoat) that you can borrow to get you through. If you're going to need to wear huge socks, you're probably going to have to buy a pair of gigantic shoes for the duration. A basic winter maternity wardrobe could include:

1 fancier dress
1 skirt
2 pairs black pants
4 pairs opaque black stockings
gigantic sweater
maternity jeans
2 maternity-size bras—maybe 1 pale and 1 black
gigantic cotton underpants

summer or the tropics

Please, just forget that polyester was every invented. Go for cotton, or microfiber or a rayon if it's the cool, floaty kind. Corner a big guy and confiscate all his T-shirts and shirts. A basic summer or tropics maternity wardrobe could include:

1 fancier dress
1–2 everyday gigantic dresses
large T-shirts
large men's shirts
2 maternity-size bras—maybe 1 pale and 1 black
loose maternity pants
gigantic cotton underpants
shawl, wrap, or giant sweater for cold evenings:
use a horse blanket if necessary

undies

⑥ The most important word on panties is cotton.

⑥ Undies can be worn under the belly, if you like a bikini style; or if you find up-to-the-waist styles more comfortable, you can probably just buy bigger sizes of your favorite brand—if or when these become tragically inadequate, you may need to invest in maternity underwear.

⑥ Women who have bad backs, are overweight, or are carrying twins may be told by their doctor to wear a maternity girdle or abdominal support to give some extra support late in the pregnancy. Maternity girdles should not be designed to make your stomach look smaller.

⑥ Real tights usually just don't fit at all as you progress in size. But why doesn't anyone make matte-black opaque maternity tights that don't fall down so you don't get that sagging gusset thing happening? Until they do, you could take a tip from Superman and wear your underpants OVER your tights to keep them up.

shoes

Yes, your feet are getting bigger—first, they're probably puffed up with extra fluid (and if you go on a plane they puff up like blow-fish) and, second, they're probably broader because of all that extra weight you're carrying. The ligaments in your feet are softer and stretchier than usual, so your feet will "spread" and well-fitting, comfortable shoes are essential.

⑥ Your feet may end up one size bigger permanently. You may want to wait and see before buying lots of hideously expensive new shoes.

⑥ If you wear socks, buy thin ones or stocking socks.

⑥ Buy a new, larger, all-purpose, flat-heeled pair of shoes to "live in" for the duration—many very pregnant women wear tennis shoes. Or pop a couple of rowboats on your feet.

Average approximate fetus length this week from head to butt

| in | 1 | 2 | 3 | 4 | 5 |

what's going on

Probably by now you will have felt the baby move, but maybe not. It's usual to laugh or cry. Doing both at once is perfectly fine. It might still be too early for anyone else to be able to feel the movements from the outside. For a while, it's your little secret bond.

The fetus puts on more muscle and tests it out by moving around. One book says your baby is as heavy as "a medium-sized Spanish onion" (do let me know if you find a Spanish onion weighing 11 ounces). The skin's sebaceous glands (needed, of course, to make pimples later) become active and make the oily stuff called vernix caseosa that covers the skin. It's the fetus's do-it-yourself wetsuit made, disgustingly enough, of fatty material and dead skin cells. (If that doesn't make you feel sick, how's this: doctors say the coating looks like cheese.) Vernix caseosa waterproofs the skin against the amniotic fluid and protects the fetus from scrapes when it bangs into the wall of the uterus. Weight: about 11 ounces.

7   8   9   10   11

DiARY I'm not depressed any more but I still haven't felt the baby move and I'm sick of all these books saying I should have. It makes me really anxious. I feel very cheated about it not kicking and really cross with the books for making me feel like a freak because I haven't felt "the quickening."

Beck says, "You have felt the baby move, but you just don't know you have. You probably thought you were going to fart or something." How romantic.

We go out to dinner and I have two glasses of French champagne and am so sloshed I sleep for 11 hours and only go to the bathroom four or five times. Remarkable.

Feeling suddenly bigger and paradoxically less fat. Probably because it all seems like it's out the front there, now. I really feel like I'm carrying weight, though—when I try to run, this galumphing, hilarious big tummy precedes me like a big beer belly. Matt says soothing, private things like, "You are *not* a fat old cow. You are the Tummy Princess."

Suddenly feel connected to other mothers a bit—certainly more than I ever have before. Not all mothers. Well, obviously. Not Pamela Anderson or Madonna or anything.

I saw Peter X. in the street today. Nothing like the wildly startled look of an old boyfriend who's about to say, "Hi, you look well," and then has to restrain himself from fainting as he realizes you're pregnant and he doesn't know what to say. His eyes rolled around in his head like the eyeballs of a rabid squirrel—lots of white. Poor thing. I suspect that just for a split second he thought it might have had something to do with him—until he came to his senses and realized that 6 years' gestation is probably pushing it.

Yesterday I paid for all my literal slackness in not doing my pelvic-floor exercises. I sneezed and wet myself. Not a huge gush, but enough to make a tiny splash on the floor. Luckily I was standing on the wooden floor at home.

When I sneezed Matt said, "You look absolutely mortified."

"Well, I just peed," I explained helpfully.

I am also having a recurring dream that I'm having an affair with a freelance sausage maker. I wonder if freelance sausage makers mind if you wet yourself.

My old friend Luke and his wife, Fatimah, call to offer a stroller. Excellent. Uncle Stan insists on buying the crib even though he will no doubt complain for 6 weeks about how much it cost and express the view that the baby should be sleeping in a hammock in the open air dressed in a robe knitted from chamomile or something.

Marg's getting on in her pregnancy now. She just called to say she was in the shoe shop and a woman told her she had good posture. Marg, completely vague and stuffed full of pregnancy info, meant to tell the shop assistant that's because when she walks she "leads with her sternum," the breastbone. Unfortunately what she actually said was she "leads with her perineum," which is the area between the vagina and the anus. No wonder the shop assistant looked startled.

Marg's not putting on enough weight and I've got plenty extra. We're considering a transference.

info

weight gain

Weight gain is an important part of a healthy pregnancy. You'll find pregnancy "experts" are all over the place when it comes to saying how much weight you should gain. The right weight gain for you is different from the right one for somebody else (you know, depending on your height, weight, and body frame when you became pregnant, and whether you give a care about it). The ranges nominated for a one-baby pregnancy vary from 25 pounds to 45 pounds. Many slender women put on 40 to 60 pounds during pregnancy and then lose it again afterward.

About a third of the weight gain is baby, placenta, and amniotic fluid; the rest is new bits of you—increased blood volume, breast growth, fluid, and fat. The body needs to build up stores of fat during pregnancy, which is then used in breastfeeding. The weight you gain will probably go something like this:

baby, placenta, amniotic fluid: 10 pounds
increased size of uterus: 2 pounds
increased breast size: 1 to 2 pounds
increased blood: 2 pounds
retained fluid: 6 pounds
increased fat and protein stores: 6 pounds

Most of the weight gain is in the fourth to the seventh month of the pregnancy.

At the birth you can lose up to 24 pounds at once, and in the days following, the excess fluid will also be lost through sweat and urine.

You will probably weigh yourself every time you visit the obstetrician or midwife, and they may give you advice on diet if they think you are gaining too much or too little.

Your obstetrician or midwife will be on the alert for any rapid increase in weight during the last 10 weeks of pregnancy, which can be a sign of preeclampsia (see the info in Week 31). Some other factors associated with too much weight gain in pregnancy are diabetes, high blood pressure, excessive juice intake, and uncontrollable Haagen Dazs addictions.

more info on weight gain

 What to Eat When You're Expecting by Arlene Eisenberg, Heidi E. Murkoff, and Sandee E. Hathaway (for details and full review see More Info on Eating and Supplements in Week 2). (They're awfully strict.)

See also Eating and Supplements in Week 2 and Exercise in Week 15.

your record

Time capsule for your child:
What's in the news this week?

What are the most popular songs? (By whom?)

What are the most popular films? (Starring whom?)

What outfit is the height of fashion right now?

WEEK 21

what's going on You could start to get heartburn and indigestion. Get used to people judging your size—"You're not very big for 21 weeks" and "My goodness, that's enormous!"—sometimes on the same day. This could be a good time to spend a day with a friend or friend-of-a-friend who has a baby under 2 or 3 months old, just to get a feel for the future.

The fetal eyelids are still fused closed (until week 27), but the fetus can hear sounds from within and outside your body. The brain has been developing very quickly, but its surface is still very smooth, not like the textbook pictures of adult brains we're used to. Weight: about 14 ounces.

You could catch stingrays in my underpants

DiARY I have new moles and skin tags everywhere. It's like my skin is hyperactive and throwing out extra bits wherever it can. Basically, I'm getting extra tags and moles in every area I already have them, plus a whole new bunch of tags under each breast.

My hair also appears to be attempting an Afro at every available opportunity. It seems to be growing faster and getting thicker, but perhaps this is an optical illusion.

My tummy's sticking out about where the rest of the world used to be, so when I squeeze through to get out of the elevator at work and automatically calculate I've got a 3-inch clearance I actually rub myself against someone, who starts to look very frightened at the idea of being groped by a pregnant woman.

Young men look me up and down in the street, and when they realize I'm pregnant there's this look of panic that crosses their face and they quickly swerve out of my way. It makes me want to rush over and get them in a vicelike grip and scream: "The baby's coming! You'll have to do something!" I think most of them would faint dead away or just run.

I was standing on the street the other day waiting for the lights to change, and just as they did a beaten-up Toyota pickup stopped and a guy with dreadlocks and a cowboy hat stuck most of his body out the window and started shouting, and then the driver was honking his horn and cat-calling, so I started rubbing my big tummy up and down, pulling up my dress and vamping across the road—because of course it was some guys from Matt's work falling about laughing. You should have seen the looks on the faces of the other drivers waiting at the lights: like, this used to be a bad area but now it's just *disgusting*.

Shopping with Aunt Peg. Thank God no horror stories, although she does tell me encouragingly at some length that ALL first babies cry CONSTANTLY and wriggle all the time and drive their parents mad, and the parents *never* get any sleep, and this is the inevitable fault of the parents, who are necessarily inexperienced and tense so make the baby tense. Quite serene, this shopping caper.

See a small child in a clothes shop and say "Hellooo" in exactly the same tone Aunt Peg uses. Reel back in horror and hope I won't automatically start trying to feed small children gray ground beef on rice and boiled pork chops four nights a week. A few minutes later say "Peekaboo" to another strange child just as if I am channelling Aunt Peg, who is at that moment looking at a pink floral suit and saying, "This is lovely, dear, unless it's a boy." (She is very worried about cross-dressing babies.) The child seems to take it rather well and in the jaunty manner it was intended.

Shopping for baby clothes is actually just like being size 10 in a shop for grown-up women where all the sizes are 4 and 6. Everything's teeny tiny. Except there are slightly more snap fasteners at crotch level than usual. When shopping for myself I can still go into a shop and say, "Yes, I'll have one of those in size ginormous, thank you." If they have them. At this stage you could catch stingrays in my underpants.

Anyway, back to baby gear. Some kids' clothes are $50 a piece, even $100 a throw, for something that they must grow out of in a nanosecond. I'm thinking I might just coat my child in Vaseline to keep it warm. There are T-shirts and rompy suit things you can buy with "Baby" written on the front—you know, in case you think you've given birth to a ferret, or you get confused and start dressing your bedside lamp. "No, that's right, tea cozy on the teapot, T-shirt on the BABY."

And there are these hair bands with flowers on that go around a baby's head, and basically they're used on a baldy baby to indicate that it's a girl. Oh, say it loud and say it proud: "The kid's bald."

People keep asking me if it's going to be a boy or a girl and I say, "Yes, I believe so. So I've been led to understand. But we're not fussy. We're just hoping for a life form of some description." They say, "Well, you should find out so you know what kind of clothes to buy for the baby." I'm like: Is it going to matter? Is somebody going to accuse a 4-month-old child of cross-dressing? "You perverted infant, you're dressing like RuPaul—get a hold of yourself!!"

And sometimes people ask, "What are you hoping for?" "A giraffe. They're up running around the paddock an hour or so after birth and starting to feed themselves."

If you don't know much about babies, the sizes are an eye opener. They start at "preemie," followed by 0–3 months, but when I say that seems so big the sales assistant shows me a doll that's the size of a 3-month-old baby and it could play receiver for the Green Bay Packers. There's no way something that big is going to come out of me without some kind of major rearrangement of the laws of physics. So 0–3 months it is—about the size of one of those gowns starlets wear to the Oscars, in fact.

I'm feeling much better, but still sleeping up to 10 hours a night easily. The whole food thing is weird. I still eat when I'm hungry but nearly hurl at the sight or smell of any slight sliminess, like green leafy things more than a few minutes out of the ground. I can't go to the market with Matt anymore because I go green the minute I smell the delicatessen section and have to go outside.

I watched a TV documentary on British comedian Spike Milligan and was astonished to hear that after they divorced he refused to let his wife ever see their children: that's what the law allowed then because she had left him, even though he was a manic-depressive alcoholic. He now says he was an unfit father. His kids talked about how they used to write letters to fairies and leave them in the garden, and Spike would write back tiny, enchanting letters and they really believed there were fairies, well into their teens. It sounds lovely, a man trying to make his children's world so beautiful. But then his son sadly describes how completely ill-equipped this made him for the real world. Oh, who'd be a parent?

We're off to Matt's work function. Matt is given a gardener's achievement award (a very nice shovel), and his colleague Brenda makes a speech in front of the entire workforce of the nursery chain stores about how his extra work is really appreciated, especially as his "wife" (apparently that's me) wouldn't appreciate him working on weekends with women in skimpy shorts (no, I really think lady gardeners should wear crinolines), but I had mounted the best strategy and got him pregnant.

I spend a good half an hour restraining myself from wrestling her to the floor and strangling her with a tablecloth.

About sixteen people handle my stomach without asking. Only one, Trina, asks whether she can. Her baby is a year old and she tries to sell me her cousin's stroller. Crushed to hear we are already strollered up on a promise, she changes topics by looking at me critically.

"How are you going with your weight?" she asks, swaying in the wind on her go-go boots.

"Oh, stacking it on, thanks," I say cheerfully.

"Don't do what I did. I got up to 175 pounds."

I break it to her gently. "I'm already 175 pounds."

"OH MY GOD! I've finally lost it all."

"Breastfeeding?" I ask.

"No, it's harder than that," says Trina. "As soon as I stopped breastfeeding, I started starving myself and eating junk food. But I'll have to start eating properly again to set a good example for the baby." Fat chance.

At Lucretia's party that meat-faced old drunk Michael F. comes up and tells me loudly I'm the last person he expected would ever get pregnant. I suggest he take a long look at Boris Yeltsin.

"Babies love me," he says. "I don't know why, but when they get a bit older they reject me."

"Maybe it's because you smell like a bottle of mixed sherry and urine," I don't say. More advice about how to get them to sleep from a man with four children by five different women, who thinks a hearty breakfast is a bottle of stout and a packet of Camels.

Today's newspaper says a new study shows that unborn babies can hear at 20 weeks. I hope Cellsie didn't get a load of Brenda's speech. Mind you, I'm really not sure about the research methods in some of these surveys that provide quotable statistics. Ten pregnant women listened to one music tape in the twentieth week of pregnancy. Two to 3 weeks after birth, the babies kicked less when those songs from the tape were played.

Well, this is just not enough information. Were the babies forced to listen to Garth Brooks, Celine Dion, or Mating Calls of the Lesser Yak? Couldn't the lack of kicks have been incredulity?

info

at work

In a healthy pregnancy and a healthy workplace there is no reason why you shouldn't keep working for as long as you want to and your doctor and human resources department agree, especially because the money will come in handy. How close to your due date you work will depend on how you feel.

Most women value some time alone before they begin the horror! the horror! Oops. The extremely rewarding and divinely bondworthy, magnificent experience of childbirth and caring for a newborn baby. It's common to take maternity leave for at least the last 2 weeks of the pregnancy, and longer if you can afford it. You'll probably feel really tired and uncomfortable in the last few weeks. Resting well, exercising gently, eating right, and thinking serene thoughts during the last weeks of the pregnancy certainly won't hurt.

From week 32 your heart, lungs, and other vital organs are working really hard and getting more and more squished up by the growing uterus. The strain on your back, joints, and muscles is increasingly intense, and you might be spacey a lot. Not to mention that by week 36 (or earlier) that baby head bouncing on your cervix can make you swear and jump around as if you've suddenly developed Tourette's syndrome: not a good look during a meeting.

If your job requires a lot of standing up, working in the last few weeks can get really difficult. Even a desk job can become hard. You might just want to lie on the couch and read magazines or watch videos.

If your job has you on your feet more than 4 hours a day, you should talk to your employer about your pregnancy. By week 24 you may need to move to a desk job, have shorter shifts, work from home a few days a week, or stop working. Standing for many hours a day at work and/or a long commute can be risk factors for preterm labor. You may need advice about your rights from your labor union.

Other work conditions that should be discussed with your doctor are exposure to possible teratogens—substances or environmental factors that could harm your baby (see the info in Looking after Your Embryo and Fetus in Week 4)—work that involves lots of lifting, carrying, or bending, or shift work, which can upset sleep and eating patterns.

Being pregnant at work should probably be dealt with like any other personal issue: don't blab everything to everybody, especially gossipy people and ones who couldn't care less and drop off for a nap at the first sign of the word "trimester." This will also allow you to feel more professional for the time you are there and when you come back from maternity leave.

Regardless of what the law requires of them, managers can vary dramatically in how they view the whole deal of pregnancy and maternity leave. Bosses in some large companies have done cost-benefit research and realized it's cheaper and smarter to give valued employees leave, then welcome them back with flexible working hours, than to drive them out and start training new people (who may also get pregnant). Other bosses try to fire you as soon as they find out: this is illegal.

◎ While you're busy being your same old reliable, efficient self, you might really be feeling very different, hiding how you feel, and worrying that you might overlook something important. Here are some suggestions that might help.

◎ Keep a stash of healthy snacks at work, which are useful for keeping your blood sugar up and nausea at bay during the first trimester, and for general nutrition the rest of the time.

◎ Make yourself comfortable. Put your feet up when you can. Sit rather than stand. Practice squatting for labor during private moments. Have regular walks and stretches if you're bent over a desk for much of the day. Drink plenty of water. If you feel really tired, use your lunch hour to sleep in a spare office, arranging to have someone wake you up at the end of the break. If you do this, don't forget to make time to eat.

◎ Take it as easy as you can. Bring work home, or go home for a snooze if you can.

◎ If work is stressful, try yoga or meditation classes and learn some good relaxation techniques.

◎ Keep the best work schedule you could imagine and religiously consult it every morning. Make lists. Invest in Post-it notes for reminders. Get color-coded folders. Get other staff pals or an assistant to remind you of things, including "Go and have lunch."

If you think you're being discriminated against, check your rights with your union, lawyer, or government departments dealing with employment.

your record

Is being pregnant affecting your work? If so, how?

Describe your job or what you do all day. (Your child
will be interested to know eventually.)

what's going on

You may have back pain, cramps, varicose veins, vivid dreams and feel strangely calm. Nearly everyone puts on the most weight in the second trimester. Of all the weight you put on, a relatively small proportion is the weight of the actual baby. The rest is stuff you need such as blood, amniotic fluid, larger bosoms, necessary fat stores, and, um, cheesecake.

Downstairs there may well be some exhibition somersaulting going on. The inner ear has reached full size. There are now eyebrows and head hair (unless you've got a baldy baby). The lungs are starting to produce stuff called surfactant, a detergentlike substance that will help them to function properly by keeping them expanded after a breath. Weight: about 1 pound.

Average approximate fetus length this week from head to butt

in   1   2   3   4   5

EK 22

fig (a) doing pelvic-
floor exercises

fig (b) not doing pelvic-
floor exercises

DiARY My horoscope this week says: "Dating is invested with potential. Those who are pair-bonded ought to beware sudden attractions to deeply inappropriate types." In my case, I presume, this would mean . . . anybody else in the entire universe.

Matt talks to all the men at work about weird things their wives do when pregnant. I don't have enough people to talk to about this stuff. Most of my friends who aren't childless have forgotten what it's like to be pregnant. Even a lot of my lesbian friends (or as my niece Seychelle calls them, ladies who love ladies) who want to have kids haven't got around to working out how yet. We are about to leave the baby-free zone.

I've been organizing a cloth diaper service for Marg for when she gets out of the hospital with the new baby. I've been sending out a form letter to all our friends.

Dear Friends,

As you may have noticed, Marg Anderson is about to have a baby any minute now. Possibly at this very moment. What you may not know is that newborn babies need their diapers changed up to sixty times a week.

Yes.

Horrible, isn't it?

To help deal with this rather confronting fact, we have organized Marg a gift account at ABC Diaper Service—which will deliver clean diapers (and take away the other kind) each week, as soon as she gets home from the hospital. (She has expressed a firm wish to receive a gift of diapers rather than flowers, which will only make her sneeze.)

You might like to contribute a week's worth of diapers ($28.50) yourself or as part of a cartel. Please fill in the enclosed coupon, add a check, and send it straight to ABC Diaper. Marg's account number is 62240. Don't forget to add your name to the coupon so Marg will receive a card with your name on it.

Love, Maddie

I am prostrate with exhaustion and self-admiration after such efficiency. Then I realize I forgot to put stamps on the letters.

This not-feeling-the-baby-move business is getting embarrassing. Beck, with absolutely no tact in sight, tells me I'm a "bit remedial." She assures me again that I have felt the baby move but haven't realized it, and she tells the story of a fat woman who came into the ER when Beck was a nurse.

The woman was complaining of terrible, sudden, intermittent abdominal pains. (You know what's coming, don't you? Well, she didn't.) The ambulance told the nursing staff the pains were coming at regular intervals and were probably labor contractions, although the woman kept saying she wasn't pregnant. Beck said to her, "But haven't you felt the baby move?" "It's just gas," the woman said, shortly before being joined by her offspring, whom she regarded with some astonishment.

I've popped into Beck's clinic, after another visit to the chiropractor, to see if I'm in early labor or just constipated. What a glamorous job she has.

"I'm not giving you a laxative without feeling what's going on," she says. "Otherwise you might be having a baby instead of a poo."

Charming.

Speaking of gas, am nearly crippled by it in the babies' department of a gigantic department store this afternoon, and have to walk around bent in half and rubbing my stomach. People look rather concerned but I can hardly announce: "It's all right, move along, I think I just need to do an enormous FART."

Once again some of the baby clothes have Paris couture prices, and although I am careful I end up spending $150 on small hats, onesies, cotton jumpsuity things and oh, all right, a couple of expensive cute things like a red denim jacket and matching leggings. Bought a few light blue items. Not because I think I'm having a boy but because that pale pink makes me feel queasy.

I think it's better if I stay out of babies' and children's wear departments. It will be cheaper, and I don't want to end up with a child resembling anything remotely like those demented-looking blond children with bowl haircuts you see in glossy kids' wear brochures, dressed in velvet frou-frou sailor suits with matching bow ties, looking like their parents would have conniptions if they got dirty. I'm thinking of dressing Cellsie in a plastic raincoat from dawn till dusk and just hosing him or her down before bedtime.

info

skin

A whole lot of stuff happens to your skin when you're pregnant. Everything is working overtime, generally resulting in more oil, sweat, and pigment (coloring) being produced. More blood is flowing closer to your skin, making it warmer; and increased oil gland secretions, giving skin a shinier appearance, add to the pregnancy glow. Retained fluid can give the skin a fuller, smoother appearance than usual. Necessary fat stores mean more cellulite on buttocks and thighs for the duration.

It depends on the individual: although many women find their skin looks better than ever during pregnancy, some may be prone to pimples or acne, while others may find themselves with dry, scaly skin. Estrogen slows down oil production, but progesterone promotes it—and they are both very active during pregnancy. Most skin changes, including some skin tags, are temporary, but some are permanent: you may end up with darker nipples forever; a few more moles and stretch marks will stay, but they'll probably fade to be hardly noticeable unless you run around in the nude under fluorescent lights.

pigmentation changes

Pigmentation changes, also known as melanin or color changes, are caused by increased production of melanocyte-stimulating hormone (MSH), which acts on the cells that affect the color of your skin. These changes are usually more obvious on dark skin. The theory is that darker nipples make it easier for breastfeeding babies to find them. If you have fair skin and red hair the changes will probably be slight.

linea nigra

The dark line called the linea nigra, which divides your tummy into halves along the site of the stretching rectus muscle (from your navel down to the top of your pubic hair), often appears by week 14, though sometimes not until weeks later. (The line is actually there before pregnancy—imaginatively and inaccurately called the linea alba, the Latin for "white line"—although it's not particularly noticeable on any skin color.)

The area around and inside your navel can also become darker. So can existing freckles and moles; and the skin under the eyes and arms, between the thighs, and of the genitals may also be noticeably darker during pregnancy. Some pregnancy experts say the vagina turns purple. But who's game to look? It doesn't matter what color it is. (Tell a lie. Lime green would be a worry.) Oh, let's just take their word for it.

irregular patches

Irregular patches of slightly different-colored skin might turn up on your face; these are called chloasma or, by doctors who used to watch *Zorro,* the "mask of pregnancy." The patches are dark in women with light skin and light in women with dark skin.

Folic acid deficiency is linked to color change in the skin. Exposure to the sun will intensify changes such as the face patches. A hat and a 15+ sunscreen will protect you.

stretch marks

Stretch marks that look like thin pink, red, or purplish lines on pale skin, and paler brown lines on dark skin, are the result of collagen fibers in the skin tearing and breaking. They can happen on breasts, tummy, thighs, and bottom. (The same hormone that makes ligaments relax during pregnancy, relaxin, also decreases the amount of collagen in the skin fibers, making them more fragile.) After pregnancy, stretch marks gradually fade to silvery lines in the skin, usually barely noticeable.

You can't stop or heal stretch marks, but as they are caused by the skin being forced to stretch a lot and quite quickly they are generally worse in cases of rapid, excessive weight gain. How many you get and how quickly they fade will largely be determined by the skin and body type you inherited. Some skins have more elastin and collagen than others.

Gradual weight gain may help to minimize stretch marks, and a good diet that includes plenty of protein and vitamin C will help keep skin in a generally healthy condition. Many people swear by vitamin E cream, but there's no scientific research that proves it helps, and many women who use vitamin E cream still get stretch marks. Using a basic lotion once or twice a day on your belly can't hurt, and may make the stretching more gradual.

skin tags

Skin tags are little extra bits of skin that often develop in places where there is some friction, such as the bra line under your breasts, or under your arms. They are caused by small areas of skin getting overactive. Sometimes they disappear a few months after birth, sometimes you've got them forever (but dermatologists can remove them). Guess you'll just have to wait and see what happens to yours.

visible veins

Some people develop spider veins: threadlike, wiggly red lines, usually on the cheeks. They are small broken blood vessels caused by rapid dilation and constriction of the blood vessels when circulation increases during pregnancy. Blue lines under the skin, on the breasts, and on the tummy just show some of the extra blood you're carrying. They will often go away after the baby arrives. Bulging varicose veins in the legs can be painful. Your doctor can tell you how to avoid them (usually: put your feet up when you can and wear special support tights). They may eventually disappear or in severe cases have to be surgically removed. If varicose veins become red, tender, and warm, notify your doctor to have a blood clot ruled out.

rashes and spots

Heat rashes can be caused by the combination of increased circulation, body temperature, sweating, and skin friction in pregnancy. Rashes might cause itchiness. It may help to dress in cotton clothes that allow good ventilation and to wash using a non-soap alternative or special oil (ask your pharmacist).

Red spots sometimes appear on the face, arms, torso, palms, and soles of the feet. These too are caused by increased blood flow through dilated vessels and go away after pregnancy.

Some medications for acne and psoriasis can be very dangerous to the developing fetus. Discuss alternative treatments with your doctor. Conditions such as eczema and psoriasis often improve during pregnancy.

what's going on

Your bladder is getting squished up even more, so you may need to pee more often. You might feel occasional uterine contractions (or they may not start for weeks, or you might not ever experience them).

Average approximate fetus length this week from head to butt

in   1   2   3   4   5

The fetus is growing like gangbusters, and the brain is maturing. Some researchers believe the fetus has started to think. Others, to be safer, say we can't really tell when this happens, and it may be much later. (And anyway, it's probably just stuff like "Gee, I like to suck things" and "La, la, la, whatever" or "It's a bit wet in here, innit?") The skin is growing very quickly, but there's not much fat yet developed for plumping up underneath it, so the skin looks a bit pruney. Weight: about 1¹⁄₄ pounds.

7   8   9   10   11

Diary

Just ate entire block of chocolate. Feel sick. This won't stop me from having lunch, mind you. By this stage I find I am in need of some even more simply enormous underpants. They are the kind of thing you could wave if you were surrendering. Later I might recycle a pair as a duvet cover. I find it is infinitely more soothing not to think about the size of my butt. I also picked up a bargain—a free pair of socks with every pair of maternity tights! Some bargain—the whole package was $20 and the tights ran when I looked at them sternly.

The only time I can get a sense of weightlessness is in the bath. I'd rather be swimming, even if I did resemble the opening sequence of *Free Willy*. But the public pools are infested with some hideous staphylococcus, germy thing that's front-page news. The reports include a hideous diagram of minute quantities of "fecal matter" floating around public pools and spreading the bug. Not for me, thanks. And the sea is too cold to swim in at this time of year unless you're one of those 80-year-old fanatics with elaborate floral bathing caps.

Marg's baby has arrived. She's a very beautiful girl with gigantic feet and no name, but never mind that: Marg did the whole labor as Warrior Woman without painkillers!

She had a trainee nurse who made her push too early— apparently the nurse thought the distension of the vaginal wall caused by the pushing was the baby's head! Marg's vagina, by this stage, was looking like it had been thoroughly beaten up. Poor Marg was very happy to see Dr. Herb, who marched in, terribly calm, put a suction cup on the baby's head, and pulled it outta there. He had to give her an episiotomy, so she has heaps of stitches. She said she was in shock afterward and thought she'd rather die than ever do that again, but a few days later she'd kind of forgotten.

Marg has stories of pushy nurses coming in at all hours and passing the baby around as if she were a football, which unsettles her. So she's told them all to bug off and will only let in the nicer nurses. She had the "baby blues" on day 4 when the real breast milk came into her breasts, but she reckons it wasn't too bad—she just let herself cry all day without feeling weird about it. She looks terribly glamorous and serene in her silky nightie, and the baby seems to be an old hand at the breast.

Marg's "at home" ensemble reminds me I don't have anything like it. I go straight to a department store to get myself a nightie and robe because a T-shirt, hiking socks, and an old coat obviously will not do. I also try to buy a back-supporting maternity-girdle-type thing. But when I mention the girdle, the sales lady asks sternly through lips, pursed like a cat's butt, "Has your doctor told you to get one? They're not recommended these days. Have you told your doctor?"

"I don't want one to hide my stomach, I want it to support my back."

"I see," she snapped. "We haven't got any."

What a ninny.

Boy, do I have this Nesting Thing really bad. All afternoon I daydream about moving the furniture. Why can't I live in a minimalist house like the ones in *Vogue Apartments* magazine? Pout for a while. I collect more boxes to put things in and cut out magazine articles that introduce a new verb, de-cluttering.

Thank God I am removed from the house by the necessity to travel and do a bit of promotion for the new fashion line. Realistic sizes are flavor of the month, but you watch—by summer every other fashion house will be back to grown-up persons jigging about in toddler-sized clothes. I have to do an interview at NPR's *Classical Music Show,* to publicize the new line. The offices are so posh that as I'm eating a muffin out of a paper bag while I'm waiting to go in, somebody comes and gives me a plate so I won't "have to be a savage."

I'm supposed to say in the interview why I've chosen these bits of classical music—and I don't even know what they are. I got them all off this relaxing CD that my beautician plays while I'm having a facial. So the interviewer's going, "And why is this passage by Debussy a favorite of yours?" and I just take a punt and say, "Look, it's got a lot of piano, and if you're in the bath you can go underwater to wash off the shampoo, come back up, and not feel like you've missed anything."

And then the interviewer says: "And you're pregnant. We had another pregnant lady in a while ago—or maybe she was breast-feeding, I can't remember."

I say, "Well, did you see her bare bosoms? If you saw her bare bosoms, she probably had passed the pregnancy stage."

Being in a huge city is really no fun in this condition. The line for a taxi at the airport is 200 people long and full of business people who look at you as if you're an alien pregnant person and never offer to help with your luggage.

And seven times out of ten when you *do* get in a taxi you're totally at the driver's mercy. Either they will not speak to you at all. You say, "I'd like to go to Fifth Street, please." Silence. "Do you know where it is?" Silence. "Do you have a pulse?" Silence. So you just sit back and relax, wondering if your family will ever hear from you again.

OR you get the ones where you say "Fifth Street, please," and they say, "How was your day? I'm just listening to Rush Limbaugh. I'll turn it up in the back. I'll tell you what's wrong with this country today. . . The Immigrant Devil makes work for Barney and yea through the valley of the Beelzebub the spawn of life will be transcended. Donald Rumsfeld is a communist and will burn dripping in hell for all eternity for his permissive Y-frontery. You know that, don't you?' And that's when you say: "Couldn't agree more! Just let me out at the next corner, thanks!"

Meanwhile, some states have refused to pass a law that protects the right of mothers to breastfeed in public because it is sometimes "just exhibitionism." Hear, hear. I am sick of these mothers pushing their strollers around the streets in string bikinis, removing their nipple tassels, and just flaunting themselves generally. I mean, it's too much. There are many people who don't know what a breast looks like, and when confronted with one in the street, for a split second before a baby wraps its mouth round the pointy bit, people could lose their reason!

And everybody knows that when a woman is breastfeeding, it is impossible not to be reminded of such classic films as *Debbie Does Dubbo*, *Swedish Knockers Akimbo,* and of course any movie starring

Pamela Anderson. In fact, breastfeeding is such a salacious and provocative act, I'm surprised it isn't banned altogether.

Obviously a lot of nursing mothers will pretend that they just want to feed their child to stop it from shrieking—but I think we all really know that it's just an excuse to behave like a scarlet woman and give all the guys in the vicinity a bit of a saucy come-on. Apparently when you're getting 20 minutes of sleep a day and you spend your life cleaning up somebody else's poop and you haven't had time to wash your hair for 3 weeks, all you really want to do is have sex with strange men in public places. Can't help yourself.

Some of the newspapers have gone wild with letters, including one from a member of the Breast Police who has managed to insult *everyone* by saying she finds mothers who *bottle-feed* their baby in public to be offensive because everyone must breastfeed. She's alienated all those moms who would love to breastfeed but can't. I hope her nipples rotate at night like propellers and keep her awake.

Today, I officially let myself go. I spend the entire day dressed in a burlap sack and moccasins, and I haven't washed my hair since Wednesday. I know the *Bold and the Beautiful* theme music by heart.

And I've been reading the preggers mags again. One suggests that you could hint to your partner that you were pregnant by serving him a dinner composed of veal, baby carrots, baby peas, and baby lettuce. And decorate the table with the white flowers called baby's breath. Matt, at least, being a professional, could tell baby's breath from a bunch of cauliflower, but even he's unlikely to make the connection.

The magazines are full of aerobicized chicks in high heels. I haven't done any side-lying crunches and I don't walk the length of Arizona every day. I have lifted no weights, cross-country skiing is a mystery to me, and I don't even know what an isometric abdominal is. I've only done 17 pelvic-floor exercises. This means by Fourth of July I'll be incontinent, broke, and 800 pounds. What I want to see is a few of these pregnancy magazines with women who were more than size 6 to start with and who've just had two nights of insomnia and half a black forest cake; and instead of male models, I want to see proper men looking unshaven and shell-shocked after seeing their first ballistic baby poop.

I've popped again: another growth surge in the tummy region. I popped at 4, 5, and now 6 months. It makes me go around singing the blues song by Howlin' Wolf, "Three Hundred Pounds of (Heavenly) Joy."

info

traveling

The best time for vacation travel is the middle trimester—you're probably not queasy, there's not much chance of labor starting, your energy levels are up, you're not too huge to get comfortable, and you're less likely to be mistaken for a large wildebeest in the dark.

Think twice about going somewhere hot, humid, and otherwise a frenzied-mosquito festival. Pregnancy has already raised your body temperature. As well, high-altitude destinations (over 6,500 feet) are not recommended because of the lack of oxygen for you and your baby.

Plan a trip that allows for good diet, rest, and relaxation, and always check in with your midwife or obstetrician before making any bookings. This is no time to press on with that adventure trek across the Mongolian plains on the back of a goat just because you planned it 2 years ago.

And if you are lucky enough to live in a developed country, this is probably not the time to visit a developing one. You might not be able to have the vaccinations you'll need, and you'll be exposing yourself and the baby to disease and the sort of medical care they make scary films about. If you insist on heading for regions where gastro bugs are common, pack diarrhea medication recommended by your doctor or obstetrician for use during pregnancy, and don't let yourself dehydrate.

If you travel anywhere overseas, get high-level travel insurance that includes medical costs. Ask your obstetrician about how to find a doctor at your destination who literally speaks your language. Carry a copy of your pregnancy medical records and a brief medical history, including your blood type and allergies, and your own obstetrician's phone numbers. If you have a problem, call your obstetrician at home in the States, even if you're in Burkina Faso. Worry about the phone bill when you get home.

by car
You can drive all through pregnancy as long as you don't rule yourself out for being severely spacey.

⊚ Take snacks, drinks, and a back support cushion if driving for long distances (and likewise on train trips). The only snacks you can buy in fast-food places have the nutritional content of a battered Mars Bar and three times the calories.

⊚ Stop, stretch, and have rest breaks, and don't hold back if you need to pee: make sure you stop regularly and go to the bathroom.

⊚ Put the seatbelt's lap strap underneath your belly and the sash between belly and breast.

⊚ You can sit on a folded towel for the last couple of weeks of pregnancy in case your waters break when you're driving, so the amniotic fluid doesn't ruin the upholstery.

by plane
Some airlines refuse bookings from pregnant passengers during the last weeks of the pregnancy in case you give birth prematurely on the flight. Restrictions and medical certificate requirements

vary from airline to airline. Don't think you can fox them by just turning up, either—they may make an arbitrary decision not to let you fly if you can't prove your due date with a doctor's note.

It's not safe to fly in an unpressurized aircraft when pregnant because of the reduced oxygen. Large planes all have pressurized cabins but smaller planes may not, and you need to find out about this from your travel agent. Oxygen levels can fluctuate even in pressurized airplane cabins, so if you are feeling light-headed ask the flight attendant for some oxygen.

❻ If taking a short vacation or trip, try to limit yourself to carry-on luggage to save having to wait on arrival.

❻ When booking flights, say you are pregnant and ask for an aisle seat (for access to the bathrooms and leg stretching) near the front of the plane (you can get on last, get off first, and have better air quality).

❻ Ask about food options, such as vegetarian or low-fat meals, that might be yummier and better for you.

❻ Get on at the last minute and ask an attendant to put your carry-on luggage up in the rack for you.

❻ On long flights avoid dehydration by drinking plenty of fluid—water, diluted fruit juice, or milk—but not alcohol, tea, or coffee. Bring your own healthy snacks.

❻ Take plenty of walk and stretch breaks. Elevate, flex, and rotate your feet while you are sitting, to help your circulation.

❻ Wear comfortable shoes and thin socks because your feet will swell even more than they do on a long flight when you're not pregnant, and put on support pantyhose if you have varicose veins. Puffiness may last for a day or so afterward (see the info on swelling and fluid retention in Week 28).

❻ To help get rid of fluid, take a French press, dandelion-leaf tea, and peppermint tea—in your carry-on luggage so they can't be sent to Botswana if you're going to Fangataufa. (DON'T get dandelion-root tea or coffee.) The leaf tea looks like a bag of dope without the heads and may amuse the security personnel if it's not labelled properly. Throw 2 or more large spoonfuls of the tea and 1 teaspoon of the peppermint tea in the French press and fill it with hot water; leave the tea unplunged overnight, then plunge and drink the lot at breakfast.

away from home

⊚ Take your own pillow in a black or patterned pillowcase (so it's harder to forget and leave it behind)—this will leave other pillows for propping under your tummy or between your legs.

⊚ In your handbag carry a few essentials such as tissues (you never know when your nose will run or stuff up or you'll need toilet paper), ear plugs, and an eye mask.

⊚ Don't even think about high heels.

⊚ Lighten your load as much as possible. Some marketing geniuses now make small cosmetic traveling kits for this very purpose. Cute but expensive—you can make up your own. Put all cosmetics, shampoos, and so on in tiny plastic bottles (you can buy them at pharmacies and grocery stores) or get sample-sized sachets, and take just enough for what you'll need while you're away.

⊚ Pack light, versatile clothes: a perfectly fine 3- or 4-day business trip can be accomplished with one black microfiber dress (microfiber doesn't need ironing and black won't get grubby so quickly), two pairs of tights, one pair of microfiber or cotton black pants, two T-shirts or shirts with short or long sleeves, two pairs of socks, four pairs of undies, two bras, and . . . um . . . a jacket. Unless somebody else will be available to carry your luggage *at all times*, plan to be able to have everything in a carry-on-the-plane-sized bag. Or have a small bag on wheels and ask someone to get it off the carousel for you.

You are very obviously pregnant by now so if you'd like to avoid people asking you lots of questions on your train, bus, or plane trip, read some erotic fiction with lurid book covers. You'd be surprised how much people leave you alone.

WEEK

what's going on

You may be feeling **constipated**. Changes in blood flow can mean your blood pressure **drops** and you may feel **faint**. This can happen when you lie flat on your back because the weight of the uterus can compress the big fat vein (the inferior vena cava) that carries blood from your lower parts back to your heart. If you do feel weird, stop lying on your back and you'll feel better again.

Many babies born at this stage have survived with the help of hospital **intensive care**, but this is by no means guaranteed. The biggest problem is that the **lungs** aren't really finished, so if the fetus came out early it would need help to breathe. The fetus still looks thin compared to the roly-poly Anne Geddes postcard-style baby but is starting to get plumper. Weight: about 1¹/₃ pounds.

in

1

2

3

4

5

6

7

8

Average approximate fetus length this week from head to butt

24

STRETCH PANTS

DiARY

Katie calls from the freeway to say she's just been to the county fair, where there was a "maternity ward"—a bustling pavilion full of twenty ewes, any one of which was "lambing" (that is, giving birth) at any one time while a woman on a microphone made an incessant commentary and people stood around waving flags and, depending on who they were, looking stunned (young men), completely horrified (young women), sympathetic (older women), stoical (older men), and antsy from eating their weight in cotton candy (children).

So of course last night I dreamt that it is me and a whole lot of other pregnant women in the pavilion. I am wearing baby-doll jammies and everyone else is in Laura-Ashley-style dressing-gowns. The commentator is sitting on a velour throne and saying, "Look at that woman. She can't give birth because she's wearing the wrong pajamas." I am mortified about the pajama situation, but just then the woman in the next stall gives birth to a small lamb and confides to me over the fence that she'll "make the best of it."

I wish my hair wouldn't be quite so eccentric. One day it looks like a full-on Big Hair extravaganza, and the next it lies down like a couple of bad pool players in a city pub.

I'm thinking more about the baby. The great festival of nesting continues. Rachel says every time she calls me there is another tradesperson in the house. This time it's the carpenter, Crazy Axel (he doesn't call himself Crazy Axel, but he should). Crazy Axel makes my long-awaited built-in closets in large pieces that he unloads off a trailer onto the sidewalk and then realizes none of them will fit through the door, and he has to saw them in half.

Installation brings a whole new sense of horror, with great big bits gouged out of the wall, and Crazy Axel's frank admission that he hasn't thought about how to install the heavy top pieces. At one point I offer a crane, but luckily some Swedish circus performers who are staying next door come in and climb up the wall and help guide the pieces into place. If the bottom ever falls out of the flying-trapeze market, these gals should be able to get a job at Ikea.

Crazy Axel distinguishes himself by running into the gate in his car, leaving the job for hours at a time, and walking back into the house without knocking. Finally, he says he can't finish the job because it's all too upsetting and drives away. Leaving his cell phone in the closet. Which rings in the middle of the night.

I'm still really sensitive to smells. I try to go to the market again, but one foot into the deli section and I nearly faint and throw up at the same time. Luckily I don't try Fish—my head might have rotated.

Why do I bother to make those few social calls to remind myself I still have friends? I distinguish myself by leaving parties when most other people are arriving. It's impossible to keep up my previous, nonpregnant pace—but hard to slow down to a real pregnant pace. This leaves just the uncomfortable feeling of being boring and guilty at the same time.

My brain is mush and I can't remember anything. I have stuck Post-it notes around my computer screen so many times it looks like a clown's ruff.

I'm sitting on the couch watching *Sesame Street* (practice) when I feel a sort of a feeling that could be some lunch rearranging itself, only it's too low down, and might be a fart but isn't, and come to think of it, I've felt it before. Eh-oh!

It's Cellsie! I feel intensely pleased with the world and can't help patting my tummy in reply.

People are still trying to get us to find out if it's a girl or boy. An article in the local paper asks, "Does discovering your unborn baby's gender spoil the surprise or does it allow for sensible planning?" It says three-quarters of American women want to know the gender—but I'm sure it has to do with thinking of the baby more as a person, so you'll take any info you can get. If the doctor could tell whether or not the kid was going to have a natural talent at soccer, you'd probably want to know that too— partly because there are so many unknowns and undercurrent worries that any hard and fast information can seem comforting.

Some women don't want to know the gender of their first baby beforehand. People are more likely to find out the gender of babies when they have already had a child or children. I suppose that's the one thing they are not prewarned about.

I squeeze into some old stretch pants and wear them down the street. And I do mean stretch pants. They are so thin that the tight gray pantery shows my butt crack (a fact helpfully imparted by Matt when we are two blocks from home) and threatens to simply catapult off my body at any moment. A rather narrow squeak for me, if I can use the words "me" and "narrow" in the same sentence.

info

childbirth education classes

where?

man watching birth video

Ask your midwife or obstetrician for their recommendation regarding childbirth education classes. Book a prenatal class as early as possible in your pregnancy to make sure you get a timeslot that suits you. Classes are held at hospitals, or birth centers, and are also offered by private childbirth educators, who are often midwives or nurses.

why?

The aim is to prepare you and your partner or labor support person psychologically and practically for labor and delivery. Well, as prepared as you can be if you've never done it before. And these classes are full of first-time parents. (Already-parents are probably at home having a nap.) The classes often have a couple of weeks dedicated to stuff that happens after the child is born—breast-feeding, baby care, and safety for newbie parents.

what?

Also known as prenatal classes, antenatal classes, and the horror video club, they're usually four to eight weekly sessions in the third trimester of pregnancy. Ask about the style of the class before you book in. Some are run as a series of lectures; others may have an open structure, allowing for discussion. Some offer hands-on sessions for practicing breathing and massage techniques; others may encourage the sharing of feelings about pregnancy and childbirth, or involve lying around on lumpy, brown corduroy beanbags discussing your innermost feelings with total strangers. Some prenatal classes focus specifically on fitness or yoga during pregnancy and after delivery and may be found through hospital, local sport or recreation centers, or yoga centers.

Ideally the person running the class will impartially present the pros and cons on issues such as pain relief, without saying things like, "Anyone who has an epidural is a big girlie wussbag," or "Anyone who doesn't have an epidural is a crazy feral hippie."

If the teacher seems to be going in a direction you don't like, try another teacher. Good classes should ensure you develop realistic expectations about what labor will be like, providing a balance between childbirth as a joyful, amazing event and the things that might go wrong or go against your picture of the ideal birth. Ask lots of questions: classes are there to give you the information *you* want.

Typical classes will provide information on how to recognize the onset of labor; when to come to the hospital or birth center or call in the home-birth troops; pain relief; and body positions that might help during labor. They almost always show videos of childbirth; provide a tour of a birth center or labor ward; and include advice on prenatal and postnatal exercise, cesarean section, induced labor, the partner's or labor support person's role, breastfeeding, crying babies, how to reduce the risk of sudden infant death syndrome (SIDS), and how to recognize postpartum depression. Check to make sure the classes include breastfeeding instruction. If they don't, find out about separate breastfeeding classes. The Red Cross offers child/infant CPR classes, which are a good way to be prepared in an emergency.

who?

You'll find that the pregnancy and childbirth books often talk about the various schools of childbirth theory, such as Ina May Gaskin's "natural" approach to childbirth (a progression from earlier theorists such as Dick-Read and Lamaze). In practice, prenatal classes tend to provide a combo of the most helpful elements from various schools of thought as they relate to the experience and philosophy of the birth center or hospital maternity ward.

You can go to birth classes on your own, but it makes far more sense to go with your birth support person. This makes it less likely that they'll be asking questions during the real thing such as "What happens now?" and "Can I have some of those drugs?"

your record

Spend a day with a parent and small baby.
When you've had a good rest, record your
overwhelming impressions.

Which room or corner will be converted to a nursery?
How do you plan to decorate it?

WEEK 25

what's going on

The fetus is about due to start putting pressure on your ribs and also on your digestive system. You could get pains down the sides of your tummy from now on as the uterus stretches.

The fetus looks pretty much like a baby at birth. It will definitely have developed its own sleeping patterns: usually awake when you're asleep and vice versa as your movements soothe it to sleep. (Perhaps this is why babies can be rocked to sleep once they come out.) The fetus may be startled by loud music and start bashing you when it hears a certain tune. Or maybe that's just dancing. This is a good time to play it music, talk to it, and see if you get a reaction. Weight: about 1 1/2 pounds.

DiARY I keep forgetting where I am in the middle of sentences: it reminds me of all those times recovering from endometriosis operations, when the general anesthetic seemed to temporarily wipe out most of my vocabulary. I have covered the house with a confetti of Post-it notes, and I keep paper and pencil AND a tape recorder next to the bed at night. So far I have written down really helpful stuff like "Remember the thing," and mumbled thoroughly unintelligible words into the tape recorder, then dropped it and stood on it on the way to the bathroom for the nine-hundredth time.

Matt inquires whether, now that I'm pregnant, I intend to eat his head. Turns out he has been watching a wonders-of-nature program on the TV about black widow spiders. I point out loftily that the praying mantis eats the head—the black widow eats the whole lot. Strangely, he doesn't look soothed by the knowledge that I have this detailed information.

A weird man on the bus tries to look up my skirt. I feel like saying, "Careful. You might meet someone coming the other way!" I've heard about men who are affected in an unseemly way by pregnancy, and here is the proof.

It takes some effort to think about what will happen after the baby arrives as I can't seem to stretch my mind past the concept of childbirth, but it must be done. Oh my God. It's not just that I'm pregnant; there's actually going to be another person along any minute, and they haven't even got their own room.

Actually I don't really mind if the baby spends the first few weeks sleeping in a cardboard box, but it would probably upset Aunt Peg. We have completely run out of money, but these are some of the things the books seem to think we should be purchasing:

✳ a gigantic industrial-strength washing machine.

✳ a fridge with a freezer big enough to store frozen casseroles for the weeks after the birth. The fridge we have is a legacy of the old shared-house days. That freezer is a lot more used to ever-emptying bottles of vodka and tubs of ice cream with a spoon frozen into them. Right now the freezer has only enough room for four sausages, a TV dinner, and eight Fruit Pops. Unless it has over-frosted again, and the door has frozen shut. We just *can't* have a baby, we haven't got the right fridge.

✳ a crib. I just refuse to buy something called a crib, though I might truck on down to the African crafts shop and get a woven flat basket. Quite like the idea of having a baby in a basket.

✳ muslin squares for catching spit-up. Oh for God's sake. I don't intend to go hunting for it.

✳ 56,000 diapers.

✳ a "nursery," a word which previously had connotations only of plants—will need to strip boyfriend of personal space, manhood, and shedlike environment by taking over his private room to achieve this.

✳ a "bonnet." I presume they mean hat. Or is it compulsory to get something with bobbles on it?

✳ a nursery floor covering, as in "The floor covering of the nursery should be linoleum or cork tiles." Ours is carpet. Maybe we could just throw a tarp down for the first couple of years.

✳ a dimmer switch, "installed for night feedings." Have a dimmer switch installed?! How much money do these books assume you have? What, now I have to sleep with an electrician? Give me a break. Might as well say, "Install a surround sound system with wall-sized video screen to simulate the sound and light show of the womb." We'll make do with an old lamp, thank you. Or I could park the crib near a window that lets in street light. Or duct tape a bicycle lamp to my head.

✳ a small sink with running water—some pregnancy book actually suggests you install one in the corner of the room. Oh, and perhaps a turret might be nice.

info

baby clothes

The exact quantity of clothing you'll need will depend on things such as whether you have a very vomity baby, how often you will be washing, and whether you use cloth or disposable diapers (cloth diapers tend to create more clothes washing because their "containment" is not as efficient as that of disposables).

It's not a bad idea to get your baby's clothes before you get too big to go charging around shops and bargain outlets. Here's what you'll need.

diapers

A newborn baby needs about sixty diaper changes a week on average. Later you use fewer diapers, but more goes into them. (That was delicately put, wasn't it?)

Cloth   If you choose to go the cloth route, you'll need about thirty-six diapers, depending on your washing plans. Cloth diapers made of 100-percent cotton are the most absorbent and healthy for the baby's skin. Start with the newborn size and move up as your baby grows. You can use either pull-on plastic pants or plastic pants with snaps for diaper covers, the over-the-diaper pants. Either can be machine washed. You'll need eight to ten pairs of diaper covers. Get ones with extra protection at the side against leaking. You can just throw the dirty ones in the diaper bin or washing machine, rinse, and shake off the water afterward.

Diaper wash services will deliver clean diapers and take away dirty ones, however many you need. Order the delivery to arrive a couple or three weeks before your baby is due, to ensure there is no chance of being caught without diapers if the baby comes early.

Disposables If you can, buy a more expensive, big-name brand in newborn-baby size, which despite the cost will be a good value for your money because they are much more efficient. Even if you plan to use only disposables, buy ten to twelve cloth diapers: perfect for over-the-shoulder protection after feeds and for general mopping up. You'll also be confronted with an occasional bottom so comprehensively pooey that baby wipes will get you nowhere. When this happens, dip a clean cloth diaper in warm water, squeeze out the excess and go in valiantly. Most changing pads can be covered with stretchy terry-cloth covers specifically made for covering the pads.

The worst diaper choice is cheap disposables, which are hopeless.

basic newborn-baby wardrobe
Be sure to wash all baby clothes in a mild detergent before using them for the first time, so they're not stiff or full of chemicals.

⊚ 6 undershirts.

⊚ 6 one-pieces (onesies).

⊚ 6–8 sleepers.

⊚ 2–3 pairs of cotton socks, or stretchy, pull-on, machine-washable booties—forget ribbons, forget handknits except for show, and you won't need socks at all if the weather is very hot, or if you plan to use full-length sleepers (which have feet in them) all the time.

◎ 8 blankets, usually easily washed flannel or cotton waffle weaves that are used for wrapping a baby up—they can also be tucked around the baby in a crib or stroller, and laid on a floor or table as a diaper change surface.

◎ bibs—you don't need these right away, and the number will depend on whether your baby vomits a lot, spits up (does small vomits), or drools a lot. To be honest, all babies drool a lot. At first get big cloth bibs, not plastic-backed, which are stiff and no good for wiping faces. Velcro-fastened bibs are much better than ribbon-tied ones or ones you have to pull over a baby's head. Some plastic bibs have a turned up edge for catching spills. You'll need about eight bibs once the baby starts eating solid foods (and maybe a shovel and nine bath towels). For breastfeeding, people usually just have a cloth diaper or a washcloth handy to mop up spit up.

summer or tropical baby
The baby may need sleepers with short sleeves and legs or may be more comfy with an undershirt and diaper as long as the insects are kept away.

A summer or tropical baby won't need as many blankets as listed, but you should keep a couple on hand for cool nights. Substitute a few soft, absorbent muslin or gauze squares if you like.

winter baby
The baby will need three or four outer items: cardigans or jackets are easiest to change. If you use over-the-head sweaters or windbreakers, make sure they have two buttons at the neck or are very stretchy. Fabrics such as velour, thick cotton jersey, or thermal materials are more practical than woolen knits, which are harder to wash and dry and can be itchy.

hints from mothers

◎ Buy natural fabrics.

◎ All clothes you get should be able to be soaked, machine washed, and tumble dried, if you use a dryer.

◎ Get long undershirts, even if they seem too long—the shorter ones end up looking like crop-tops. Good undershirts have really generous neck and arm holes so that you can get them on your baby quickly and easily—ones with raglan sleeves are ideal.

◎ Sleepers are so much easier to change if they have snaps that run from the neck to the crotch and right down the inside of onr or both legs of the suit. DO NOT BUY A SINGLE THING THAT BUTTONS DOWN THE BACK OR LACKS CROTCH FASTENERS. Remember, you need to go up a size in sleepers as soon as they fit snugly, or they will start to hurt your baby's feet and stop legs stretching out properly.

◎ If you buy those headbands with a bow on them for a girl baby your child will look like a demented Easter egg in a diaper.

◎ A small baby doesn't need shoes except for show (or to keep socks on). Warm, snug socks are fine—it's not going hiking any time soon.

◎ A surprising number of bonnets and hats have long cords on them. Don't buy them—they're too dangerous. In fact, don't buy anything with cords or flappy tassels or long strips of loose material—they are all strangulation risks.

◎ A very new baby hates being dressed and undressed. Choose soft, stretchy cotton or cotton-blend clothes. To help make changes quicker and less traumatic, get wide-necked onesies, for a newborn baby: easy to get over the head, and handy access to the diaper at the other end.

◎ Go to bargain places that sell seconds, but call first to see which brands they have, and why they are being sold at discount.

Small marks that will wash out are fine, but clothes likely to spontaneously combust are not.

⑥ Borrow as much as you can. If it has to be returned, keep a list! Don't ask people to lend you baby clothes—they will offer if they want to. Sometimes they are keeping their baby clothes in case they decide to have another one, and it's all too psychologically confronting to give away their supplies.

⑥ Buy or borrow the minimum number of tiny-sized clothes: they don't get worn for very long and some big babies can skip newborn clothes and go straight to the 3–6 months size.

⑥ Babies grow out of things so quickly, you could well match up with someone with a slightly bigger baby and someone with a slightly smaller baby to become part of a clothes chain.

⑥ If you don't have friends with spare baby clothes available to borrow, and you're on a budget, go for used clothes (see the Yellow Pages). Launder everything well, particularly if it has been stored in mothballs (napthaline) or camphor, both of which are poisonous, or in dry-cleaning bags, which retain fumes.

⑥ Cheaper chain stores can have very good babies' and children's wear departments: sometimes the best clothes are the cheapest because they're not fussy and made for show. At this early stage they won't need to last unless you're passing them down the line to other children. Don't overbuy, even though the clothes are so cute; your baby will grow quickly.

⑥ Used-clothing stores are good sources of knits. If need be, take someone with you who knows the difference between real wool and acrylic and buy the real wool, which is less allergenic and less flammable.

your record

What clothes have you bought your baby?

What music have you played the baby, and which songs prompted a kicking reaction?

YOUR BABY is SHOWING SIGNS OF INTELLIGENCE

what's going on
Get lots of rest and exercise. (You should also get gifts consisting of large gems, but this is unlikely.) If you haven't worked it out already, stop wearing shoes with heels, and don't do any climbing or hurling yourself about: remember your center of gravity has changed and you need to protect your tummy. You will be steadily gaining weight.

Average approximate fetus length this week from head to butt

| in | 1 | 2 | 3 | 4 | 5 |

EK 26

This coming month the fetus will really spend time putting on more fat and muscle. Each week its chances of survival outside the uterus increase as it makes more surfactant for the lungs. According to one pregnancy expert, this week in the uterus your baby "is showing signs of sensitivity, awareness, and intelligence." So if you put a little calculator in there your fetus could probably estimate the Gross National Product of Botswana. It can detect light even through its still-closed eyelids, smell (sadly for the fetus the only thing on offer is the amniotic fluid, which probably smells like a swamp), as well as hear, and possibly play the slide guitar. The baby will recognize other voices from now on: friends, Daddy, aunties, and Dusty Springfield singing "Son of a Preacher Man." Weight: about 1^3/$_4$ pounds.

Diary Are the leg cramps causing insomnia, or can I feel the leg cramps because I'm awake in the middle of the night? What a fascinating philosophical question. Beck says there are two things that might be causing sore calves: blood pooling in the veins, or lack of calcium or magnesium—in my case probably magnesium as I am taking enough calcium to turn into a tusk. For the itchy, runny nose and sneezing, she suggests a special garlic-and-horseradish dose.

"What about this gigantic tummy?"

"That will settle down in a few weeks."

My tummy is now not just a big ball out the front, but a bulge all around the sides, the supporting tissue wrapping quite tightly, like wide bandages under the skin. Not quite like love handles— too curvy to really get a grip on.

Did I mention insane heartburn and indigestion?

Pregnancy is just an absurd strain on the body, and we don't expect that anymore. We expect there to be a pill or an exercise or a mantra or a caring discussion that will alleviate "discomfort"— and "pain." Nope. It's just a pure and simple pain in the ass (and the rest) for a few months. I'm sorry, but I'm not finding this a sublimely spiritual experience. It's a deeply PHYSICAL experience.

The feeling of a baby moving must be different for everybody. Some books say it feels like gas, or feathers, or gentle patting. Sometimes I think it feels like someone's twanging a ligament as they might test out a harp string; sometimes it's like a bit of inside bongo work—all these feelings still all very low down in my tummy. Although the bump seems to start under the bozoom, the top of the uterus is actually just at navel level. All the stuff above is displaced bits making way for the uterus.

This morning's paper reports that a computer-driven baby doll is being used to help teenagers realize how much work a baby is. The baby doll is taken home from school over a weekend and is programmed to cry constantly or several times, day and night. A special sound indicates how often the diaper must be changed, and the student must decide how often the baby needs to be fed. One student who had the baby doll for the weekend said, "It really put me off having kids." You should try pregnancy, my dear.

What an incredibly unraunchy life it is: so far this week I've had half a glass of red wine (Oops. Forgot I had a bun in the oven), nine Fruit Pops and a Haagen Dazs, and some calcium tablets, and my garden is about to get its daffodils in. AND WHAT'S MORE I am becoming a stately pregnant lady and am now so considerably fattened up that that THING has happened. That THING where your thighs rub together up at the top. If I wore corduroy pants while I was walking, I'd sound like a sword fight.

I decided to check out Shirley MacLaine's pregnancy workout video, which sounds more spiritual than physical: the one in which Shirley uses a naked shop dummy with no arms and legs to explain where your chakras are. There is a lot of talk about innate spiritual reality and body fluids as they relate to creativity and the orange chakra resonating to the note D.

Shirley sits or stands around in a pink tracksuit and pink socks, and for a spiritual person she is really quite bossy and snippy. There is a lot of tinkly-dangly keyboard music. After some great kaleidoscopey patterns Shirley says: "Question your spiritual nature. Who are you? And focus on what you very much want to happen."

Shirl, I'd very much like you to explode. Shut up and have a Fruit Pop.

There must be an easier way to relieve stress, so I stay on the couch for another day and check out a wacky new-age magazine, which, sadly, turns out to be the organ of choice for people who see conspiracies in everything and an alien in every mailbox. This issue, for example, contains stories explaining how pet food is itself made from dogs and cats, and how the Cold War was a cruel hoax because the United States had given Russia the bomb plans; and book reviews of *NASA, Nazis, and JFK* and—hello, I think we've stumbled onto a mysterious connection here—*The Great Book of Hemp*. There are, however, some very impressive ads, including one for a fabulously scientific device called a Zapper, which "frees your body from viruses, bacteria, and parasites in 7 minutes!" Zappers are apparently inspired by suggestions made in a book called *The Cure for All Diseases*, which as you can imagine is a bit of a medical breakthrough. I'm surprised we haven't heard more about author Hulda Regher Clark, Ph.D., N.D.

That is not all, however. *Nexus* magazine also advertises exclusive products, including Kirlian photography cameras, which represent the energy levels of the body in a visual form, and aura cameras. The only further info is that the process is named after Semyon Kirlyian and his wife Valentina, who live in a small town in the Ukraine. Which is enough to make anybody send money.

The same company will deliver to your door some White Gold Powder: "This is a unique white powder said to come directly from gold—something which alchemists have attempted to produce for centuries. Take just one-eighth of a teaspoon under the tongue twice daily." BUT IT DOESN'T SAY WHY.

Other lovely gift and hobby ideas include building an underground library, getting a second passport, how to channel your higher self (I've never liked my higher self—she's a stuck-up cow), crapping on about guardian angels and/or interdimensional human beings, the wonders of urine treatment (make mine a Tylenol, thanks), dream control—many of these, by the way, available from a post office box in Montana—fermented living food, herbal teaology (I looked in vain for Have-a-Good-Lie-Downology), and reversing the aging process. Possibly by dying. That's enough exploring of my spiritual side during pregnancy, thank you. I'd rather have leg cramps.

info

baby equipment

You're about to enter the world of safety warnings—try to keep in mind that most babies are robust little critters, but they still need to be protected. All the baby-wrangling gear listed below needs to be safe and the best reference is the U.S. Consumer Product Safety Commission (www.cpsc.gov).

If you're going to do a lot of this shopping on foot, do it now while you still feel energetic. The major items can be bought or rented from baby-gear shops. Smaller stuff can be bought at supermarkets or drugstores. You can get second-hand baby equipment through classified ads, thrift shops, friends, and notices online. Replace any worn straps and any Velcro: there's an unofficial motto in the baby world, "One baby, one lot of Velcro."

baby seat for the car

A baby car seat is compulsory for transporting a baby in a car. A baby seat is a specially designed seat, attached by straps to an anchor point (in new cars since 2001) and further secured by a seatbelt in the backseat of the car. For older cars, you secure the seat with seatbelts. You're required to buy a restraint that complies with federal safety standards. *Consumer Reports* rates some as better than others. For babies less than 20 pounds and under 1 year old, you must use a rear-facing seat. You can get installation of a car seat checked by any car dealership, police station, or fire station.

Don't buy a secondhand one unless it's in very good condition and you know its age and history. You should never buy a seat more than 5 years old. Make sure it hasn't been in a collision/wreck.

Station wagons will need a cargo barrier to stop flying shopping bags or dogs from injuring the baby if you have to slam on the brakes. A relatively recent warning: don't leave a baby sleeping unattended in a baby seat you may have brought in from the car. Their little head can slump forward and their airway can get blocked. Most babies will rouse themselves; a few won't be able to.

baby's bed

Whether you choose a bassinet, cradle, basket, or crib for your baby's first weeks, it should meet U.S. Consumer Product Commission standards. This is no time to skimp or save money: peace of mind means a safe baby and a better sleep for you. Whatever you choose will need a firm, well-fitting mattress, two mattress protectors made of waterproof-backed fabric, and at least three sheets. You can buy fitted cradle sheets of terry cloth or flannel (it's not necessary to buy the sheets made of fine linen with ittle wuvvly la la duckies embroidered on them, which cost a bomb and would be covered in green liquid poop as soon as you look at them), or you can cut up adult bed sheets. Thin blankets or pillowcases can also be used for cradle sheets. Two or three cotton blankets that can be firmly tucked in are safer and easier to wash than a duvet, which can cut off the air supply and smother a baby. Pillows, duvets and crib bumpers are also dangerous and unnecessary. Most kids don't use a pillow until they're about two.

Bassinets, cradles, and baskets are only for young babies, so you need to ask yourself if you really need one, since your baby will be going into a crib within a few months anyway. Before you choose a baby basket (also known as a Moses basket), you need to consider whether you will want to leave your baby safely unattended in one. It's not easy to find a basket with a firm, tight-fitting mattress. And if you have it on the floor a lot (it's not safe to have it higher as it may fall), will you hurt your back lifting it and the baby?

Cradles too are soothing, but the soothing motion can be replicated by gently patting your baby in a crib, or rolling the baby in a stroller back and forth over an arm's length. (Don't leave the baby unattended in a stroller.)

Bassinets, baskets, and cradles are cozier for the first few months than a crib, even though they're not strictly necessary. A well-swaddled newborn baby can be comfortable in a crib, and a slightly older baby can be "dressed" in a quilted-cotton sleeping-bag with arms (from babies' wear outlets). Cribs can be made up at the bottom end, so there is no danger of the baby wriggling under the blankets (new babies tend to wriggle in the direction away from their feet).

Many crib designs on the market are potentially dangerous. Babies can be trapped, or injured on sharp protrusions or get stuck down between the mattress and the side of the crib. A mattress should be firm and fit snugly, with no more than a 1-inch gap between it and the crib on all sides. Other important factors include the spacing of bars, the security of a drop side, the efficiency of wheel brakes, what the crib is made of and painted with, and the position of the mattress relative to the height of the sides. Make sure you get the latest information from the U.S. Consumer Product Safety Commission for crib safety before you buy.

carriage or stroller

Technically a carriage is the huge, old-fashioned type, with gigantic wheels, that a Mary-Poppins-style English nanny would push around with the sixty-seventh Earl of Whatever inside. There are also the newer, lighter designs that can be converted into a stroller. Most people choose to use a stroller over a carriage. Some strollers have fully reclining seats like carriages. Many infant car seats are made to snap into strollers. When the baby grows out of the infant car seat, he or she can then sit directly in the stroller seat. These infant-car-seat-stroller combos are called "travel systems" by their manufacturers—parents can transfer a sleeping baby from car to stroller without waking them. Again, lots of carriages and strollers on the market are not considered safe. As well as safety, you'll need to consider cost, durability, and adaptability.

Do you need all-terrain wheels? If you live in a cold climate, make sure there are no open parts on the side through which the wind can blow, and that the carriage has a cover. If you don't go jogging or hiking you probably don't need the fancy three-wheeler. Is the carriage or stroller light and easy to fold if you are going to put it in the car or on a bus a lot? (Don't take the manufacturer's or sales assistant's word for it—fold it up and down yourself a few times in the shop.) Do you want it to convert to a stroller or will you buy one later, or do you have one lined up from a friend?

Is the carriage comfortable for you and your partner to push? Is the handle height right, or adjustable? Can you walk freely or do your feet bump into the undercarriage? Make sure it has a five-point harness for the baby, good brakes, and a shelf or basket underneath large enough to hold your diaper bag or shopping bags.

It's not safe to leave a baby sleeping in a carriage or a toddler sleeping in a stroller unsupervised for even a few minutes.

light for nighttime feeding

Either a dimmer setting for the main light in the baby's room or a small, low-wattage lamp, which provides just enough light for you to change and feed by, is useful. (Here's one theory about why nipples and areolae go darker after a pregnancy: small babies see contrasts rather than colors and can more easily spot the feeding station in a bad light.) A dim light helps to say to a baby, "It's still nighttime. Have a quiet feed, no chatting, do the business and back to sleep."

Recent research indicates there may be an association between nearsightedness and a light left on in a baby's room all night in the first 2 years of life. If you need a night light, keep it very dim and indirect.

changing table

You will be changing gerzillions of diapers, so it makes sense to do it as comfortably as possible. If you can't afford a changing table, improvise by buying a plastic-covered, hard foam changing mat with built-up sides and putting it on a hip- or waist-height table or dresser. Even if you have a changing table, one of these mats is useful to throw in the car when you're traveling or out. If you can afford an expensive changing table, go for a solid wood one. Wood ones usually have a few shelves underneath, which are very handy for diapers, a change of baby clothes, and blankets. Everything you need to change a diaper must be placed within arm's length of the changing table beforehand because you can't walk away from a baby on a changing table.

bath venue

Early on it is so much easier to wash a baby in a kitchen or bathroom sink (being careful of fixed spouts) than lugging a heavy, full plastic bath around. But if you do need a separate bath, consider buying a plastic laundry bowl or storage tub, which can be re-used.

You'll also need two or three soft bath towels. These are great for wrapping a baby in after a bath, but for drying sensitive newborn-baby creases and crannies you can also use a soft, clean cotton diaper or blanket. You can buy towels with a hood to keep baby's head warm.

For toiletries, buy a baby bath liquid or soap alternative, or an unscented bath oil; blunt-ended nail scissors; a moisturizing baby lotion; cotton balls, baby wipes or wash cloths and a water container; and a barrier cream such as zinc and mineral oil cream or other diaper rash cream. Ask around to find out what products people recommend, then buy small sizes to test on your baby.

feeding gear

You'll need nursing bras and nursing bra pads for when you breastfeed. The pads, which soak up any leaking milk before it hits your clothes, can be bought as paper-based disposables or fabric washables. Have some disposables at least in your handbag for emergencies.

A breast pump is handy for expressing milk if you're ready for a night off, your breasts are painfully full, or you need to go to work. Electric ones are better than hand pumps for expressing often; say, for going to work. You can buy or rent from pharmacies, baby-gear shops, and lactation consultants. If you're planning to leave the occasional expressed breast milk feed, you'll also need one or two bottles and nipples, a sterilizing unit (or you can just boil things), and bottle- and nipple-cleaning brushes. You can freeze portions of breast milk in special plastic bags available in pharmacies.

For bottle-feeding, you'll need six to eight bottles and nipples, bottle- and nipple-cleaning brushes, formula, perhaps a measuring cup (although most bottles have measurements on them these days), a sterilizing unit, and an insulated bottle-carrier. Bottles are supposed to be always kept very cold and then warmed just before use.

bottom re-upholstering accoutrements

A diaper bin with a lid is essential if you're washing your own diapers.

even more stuff

You'll probably find the following items useful:

⑥ a diaper bag—any big bag that has a shoulder-strap handle will do, but some are specially designed to fold out like a portable changing table. (For details of what goes in it, check out the info in Week 43).

⑥ a baby monitor—like a one-way walkie-talkie set, this is helpful if the nursery is out of earshot.

⑥ a sheepskin (also called lambswool) or two—some people like to have these under the crib sheet, or thrown on the floor or placed in the carriage for the baby to lie on. They need to be washed regularly, otherwise they can harbor gerzillions of dust mites, but can be machine washed and tumble dried.

⑥ one or two quilted or flannel baby sleeping bags—these washable, zip-up bags are very cozy in a big crib or a carriage in cold weather, but make sure you remove any dangly lace, ribbon, or drawstrings.

⑥ a baby-carrier or sling—great for comforting a fretty or crying baby while getting on with whatever else you need to do. Wearing a baby-carrier or sling is a good way to take walks or go shopping when the baby is little, though it can be hard on the back when the baby starts to stack on weight. A baby should only spend 1 or 2 hours in it at a time. Try it on before you buy it: look for well-padded shoulder straps, sturdy fabric, detachable drool bibs, a head support, and secure and easy-to-use clasps. Babies outgrow slings by 5 or 6 months, but can continue in a well-made baby-carrier with strap supports: otherwise the weight of the baby may hurt your back as they grow

❾ a safe heater—you can dry clothes in front of it if you live somewhere wet and cold. Compare the safety features of heaters on the market before you buy.

A few months further down the track you will need a high-chair, and may also want to buy a mobile, a playpen, a bouncy seat, a baby jumper, a backpack, a portable crib, and a large aircraft carrier to put them all in.

more info on safe baby equipment

Baby Proofing Basics by Vicki Lansky, Book Peddlers, Minnetonka, MN, 2002.
Enough safety hints to keep even the worry wartiest happy.

See also Safety in Help.

THE GREAT PACIFIER DEBATE

You'll find most of the baby books sternly frown on using a pacifier, especially after the baby is 3 months old. Pacifiers aren't supposed to be used automatically as soon as a baby cries. But if a baby is fed, clean, and burped and yet has got itself into a hideous, sobbing, can't-remember-why-I'm-crying-but-I'm-hysterical-now-and-can't-stop-yelling state, a pacifier is heavenly. Take no notice of what the books say; the authors aren't there to hold the baby when you're going nuts. Wait and see if your baby is like this before buying a pacifier.

If you do decide to use one, here's the huge drawback nobody tells you about. The baby may become "addicted" to it, and if so there'll be a period when the pacifier will actually make the baby cry more because when a pacifier falls out the only way a young baby can get it back in is to cry for you to come and put it in—several times a night. These weeks can be just not worth it and a good time to wean the baby off the pacifier. Eventually, some time between 5 and 10 months, a baby is able to replace a pacifier on its own, and so the "addiction" will continue.

Make sure you get the right-sized one that meets the federal standards. Replace it every few weeks, and throw it out if it looks the worse for wear with wobbly or torn bits. You'll need at least two or three to rotate them through the sterilizing process once your baby works out how to spit out the pacifier—and then to cry for it after it's hit the floor.

your record

What baby equipment have you bought?

What have you borrowed, and from whom?

List any heirlooms or toys being passed down to your baby.

What are you buying for your child to pass down to their child?

what's going on

Hurrah, you're in the third trimester. Hire a brass band: bah de bah, bah de bah. If people don't stand up for you on the bus, say, "Excuse me, I'm pregnant. Could I sit down?" About twelve people will rise from their seats as if given 140 volts up the fundament. Your moles may be getting bigger and you may have small skin tags, especially under the arms and breasts. You need a lot more fluids from now until the birth. You can forget about moving gracefully. People will not be saying, "Aren't you Audrey Hepburn?" You need to put your feet up when you can: at work, if possible on another chair—better still, make the boss massage your feet.

The fetus has grown so much it is running out of room, and it takes a little longer to maneuver about and turn upside down and sideways. Babies born now have a very good chance of surviving (they're called "viable" in doctorspeak). The fetus has been practicing breathing here and there, but from now on its breathing will become more rhythmic and constant. Folds and grooves appear on the surface of the brain, which is developing very quickly. (Of course

if the fetus is born early, all this developing will continue outside

the uterus, usually in a incubator with respirators and other

monitors attached.) Weight: about 2 pounds.

Lordy

WEEK
27

THE MAJESTIC
PROPORTIONS

DiARY It's true, you can spend an entire week in a robe, although I accessorize it differently at work. I find that when I team it with battery-operated earrings and a beehive hairdo people tend not to notice the robe. I have developed approximately sixteen billion skin tags and my moles are all getting bigger. I am looking like a currant scone, so instead of calling Cellsie Cellsie we have started to call it the Blini (a relative of the currant scone, how intensely hilarious).

Maybe I'm practicing not getting much sleep because I wake up for an hour or so every night and lie there with vaguely aching legs, listening to the blood swishing in my ears or my heartbeat in the silence. It is very disconcerting. My blood sounds like languid wobble-board music and I don't really want to be reminded of Rolf Harris in the early hours.

I have purchased a giant inflatable ball to sit on, which is supposed to be good for strengthening the back muscles. Matt immediately lies on top of it and rolls headfirst into a bookcase.

Jo rings to say she spent the first 3 weeks after her baby was born looking at him and feeling nothing, but now she adores him, and do I want some sleepers? Liz emails to say she looked at her baby for the first time and said, "Now I have to put this weird screaming creature on my breast? What would I want to do that for?" I'm grateful people are being so honest.

Matt just found out he can get 3 months unpaid paternity leave. I'm very relieved but kind of pissed off he didn't find out before. It would have saved me a lot of "what if?" thinking time. I'm getting scared about how much has to be done before the baby is born. After 2 hours' sleepless panic in the middle of the night about coping with it all, I decide to work from home: if I'm not fooling myself, I'm not going to fool anybody else. (Maybe I can get that on a letterhead.) Besides which, at the end of every day my feet smell like the world is ending—because they have swelled up to eggplant proportions all I can wear is my pair of Hush Puppies, with the elasticky bit cut.

Outrageously, Dr. Herb has gone to Paris with his wife in some sort of ludicrous attempt at a private life. I spend ages in the waiting room looking at pictures of thin people in magazines, then have to put up with another obstetrician, who while clearly competent and replete with all his marbles doesn't have the bedside manner of Herb, and indeed doesn't even help me to sit up after examining me. He tells me with a disapproving look that I have put on 30 pounds since the start of my pregnancy.

"Most people," he says, "have put on 17 to 20 by this stage." Why he didn't just call me Mrs. Blimpy I don't know.

I have a blood test after drinking a revolting sugar drink, which checks for glucose levels, anemia, and antibodies.

Afterward I go to visit Beck to say, "Help me, I'm Mrs. Blimpy."

She says, "That's crap!" (I do love a medical adviser who says, "That's crap.") "Some people put on 40 pounds when they're pregnant."

However, we agree that if I can nourish the baby and not get fatter myself, this will be a lot easier to carry around. So I must take the special pregnancy multivitamin-calcium supplements. I must stop eating Haagen Dazs, and stop bagels and cream cheese for breakfast. I must have oatmeal with some apple or half a banana in it.

"Can I have raisins in it?" I whine piteously.

"You can have four," she says.

I strike her.

Then I go out to dinner and have lemon tart with ice cream. Ya gotta live.

info

safety

The only way to childproof a house is to never let a kid in it. But you can try to make it safer.

The older the baby gets, the more danger-ous the house gets. Baby books will tell you what tricks your baby is likely to be up to next. Remember that there's a wide age range for milestones: your baby could be an early roller; your toddler could be an early climber.

As said in last week's info, every baby-relevant item needs to be safe: cribs, strollers, car seats, baby chairs, toys, changing tables, clothes, pacifiers—the lot. Remember when you are preparing the house for small persons that the most common causes of death and injury in little kids include car and pedestrian accidents—often in their own driveway—drowning, suffocation, falling, burns, poisoning, and electrical accidents.

You will need to organize:

❀ a tamper-proof cabinet for any garden poisons and chemicals, and a first-aid kit placed higher than a child on a chair or bench could reach.

❀ cupboards in which the following have been moved to a higher position—household poisons such as cleaning agents and detergents; medicines; alcohol; batteries; pesticides; mothballs and camphor; soaps and shampoos; cigarettes; matches and lighters; cosmetics and perfumes; essential oils; foods that could cause choking, such as peanuts and marshmallows; plastic bags (and go through closets to get rid of dry-cleaning bags); glasses and other breakables; objects with sharp bits—babies and toddlers can be gymnastic and inquisitive. You can also get a variety of cabinet and drawer locks to "lock" cupboards and drawers.

❀ smoke alarms.

❀ electrical circuit breakers and plug covers.

❀ no keys left in house cupboards or doors.

❀ a bathroom heater fitted high up on a wall.

❀ hair dryers kept away from water.

❀ fire screens for heaters and open fires.

❀ a water heater set to 122°F (takes longer to burn the skin than the usual, hotter setting).

❀ a stove hotplates guard.

❀ an out-of-reach kettle and iron.

⊚ appliance locks, specifically oven and toilet locks.

⊚ electrical cords that are placed off the floor and out of reach—curled cords on kettles and irons are good.

⊚ a fire extinguisher for the kitchen.

⊚ stair and doorway barriers.

⊚ a nursery with a high shelf and a toy box with a lid that is child-safe, meaning it will not close quickly and squish a child's fingers.

⊚ a pool fence with a self-latching, self-locking gate at your place and the places of neighbors (if a neighbor won't cooperate report them to the police—pool fences are compulsory), relatives, and friends—anyone who has a pool or pond. Your baby might walk before 12 months and crawl way before that. Always empty toddlers' wading pools and baths after use. Babies can drown in a tiny amount of water.

other people

Never hesitate to ask people to smoke outside the house, put down hot tea or coffee while holding your baby, support the baby's head properly when holding, and not bounce the baby up and down after a feeding. They'll probably be glad of the instruction: many non-baby-wrangling friends want some guidance.

Grandparents or older friends and relations may need a firmer hand. Practices from their own parenting days, such as not using a baby seat in a car, are unsafe. Their homes will also need to be checked.

prevention

⊚ Read the info on baby clothes in Week 25 and on baby equipment in Week 26 for safety hints.

⊚ A nursery door lockable from the outside with a hook (not a key, which could get lost) can prevent a toddler from helpfully throwing toys or food in with the baby when the baby's asleep, or tossing the baby out of a crib like a toy.

◎　Always remove bibs before putting a baby to bed.

◎　Never leave a small baby unattended with another small child, a cat, or a dog. Never put a child, a cat or dog, and food together.

◎　Sterilize anything that goes into your baby's mouth until at least 6 months old—okay, you don't have to boil your nipples.

◎　Put cribs, strollers, and baby chairs out of reach of any dangly curtain ties or blind cords, stoves, heaters, fires, and plugs.

◎　Turn all pot and pan handles toward the back of the stove.

◎　When you are traveling or at someone else's place, you might need to bring safety stuff with you and be a bit more vigilant, particularly where there are other young children and dogs.

◎　Don't leave a baby to feed unsupervised from a propped-up bottle.

◎　Don't attach a pacifier to a baby's clothes with a ribbon or string.

◎　Don't leave a baby, even for a second, unsupervised on a changing table.

◎　Never leave a baby or young child in a bath, no matter how briefly.

emergencies

Keep a contact list near the phone and add emergency numbers to your direct-dial system. The numbers should cover the ambulance (911), local doctor, and local poison control center (1-800-222-1222). Baby-sitters should be told about it. You can do an infant and child mouth-to-mouth and CPR (cardiopulmonary resuscitation) course with the Red Cross or get an instructor to come to your play group.

Add a thermometer and baby Tylenol to the family medicine cupboard and/or the baby bag. Ask your doctor when you can use the Tylenol.

more info on safety

It's No Accident: How Corporations Sell Dangerous Baby Products by E. Marla Fletcher, Common Courage Press, Monroe, ME, 2001.

Products that are not properly tested can harm babies and children. This book is an expose on the industry and names of dangerous items.

www.cpsc.gov

The website of the Consumer Product Safety Commission has a special section on recalls and warnings on faulty or dangerous products. It also has printed or Web booklets on making a safe home for your baby and kids.

Children's hospitals are good resources when it comes to safety issues: some also sell safety products. Your pediatrician or nearest children's hospital may have their own checklist.

 See the list of contacts under Safety in Help.

what's going on For you, just more of the same, really.

Your baby may be hiccuping. It will usually decide to party while you are resting or asleep. Its eyes are partially opened—quite sensibly as who would want to open their eyes wide in a fetid old swamp of amniotic fluid? The baby is now covered all over with vernix, so it looks a bit like one of those long-distance swimmers smothered in gunk. Except babies have got more brains than to try to swim from Cuba to Florida. They just hang out in the uterus growing their bodies so their heads don't look too big. Weight: about 2 pounds.

WEEK 28

DiARY

My feet hurt to walk, and my tummy's really starting to pull forward, so of course it's time to go traveling again. I'm at Fashion Week in New York.

The usual lot get all the publicity, and if anyone mentions Prada to me again I shall have to have them killed. There's nothing wrong with a lacy wisp of foam and a scrinch of lace webbing between your bosoms, but it's not like you can actually DO anything in it other than accept your best-supporting-actress-in-a-drama Emmy award. As one does.

Planes always make my feet swell up, but now it seems to work on the whole body. My fluid retention after I get off the plane at midday is clearly visible to the naked eye. Have gone quite bullfroggy around the face, and the indent marks on the ankles where the socks come up are like trenches. Luckily Beck had suggested I pack some dandelion-leaf tea, which I make at my hotel in a french press I buy in the lobby shop. The tea tastes as well as looks like lawn clippings. I get so desperate, I make it up and drink it mid-afternoon instead of waiting until morning and am peeing all night. It works, though.

People now have their routine down pat: "When are you due?" followed by "Do you know if it's a boy or a girl?" followed by "Is it your first?" I go to a very Fashion Week-y cocktail party (vodka ice pops instead of devils-on-horseback—but not for me) and meet the lead singer of Staid, who asks, "Is it exciting?" I think this a much better question and talk his ear off him until his eyes glaze over and he staggers to the refreshment tent, supported by an elfin keyboard player from a visiting Canadian band called Prince Phillip's Undies.

It's becoming harder and harder to maneuver the body around, and I am sad to say that grunting while changing positions is by no means unknown. I do it on the plane home and gross out the chemical weapons salesman sitting next to me. I find it very difficult to believe that Matt would want to have sex with me, and he admits that he doesn't want to ask because (a) I seem so tired, and (b) my body seems rather preoccupied, but he does want to have sex with me because he loves me. This is the sort of answer people should win a lounge suite for on quiz shows.

We try having sex but it is really quite an absurd proposition. It is impossible to avoid the conclusion that there are three of us involved. Well, there are. I wish I could unstrap the Blini for a couple of hours.

I can now see cellulite on my thighs without having to pinch the skin together. Matt says, "It's for a reason," and "It's temporary," and "It doesn't matter" (give the man another lounge suite, please), but if THIS is what size I am at 6 months pregnant, I am terrified to think of me at 9 months. Especially the little matter of getting it OUT.

Sometimes the Blini kicks really hard and I get a shock. "Sit down in front!" yells Matt. And quite often I am forced to move because the baby is clearly going to make the position unbearable by stretching against me somewhere uncomfortable. It's fascinating that so many women say they love to feel their baby move, but they never tell you that sometimes it's really horribly uncomfortable and sometimes it even hurts. Last night in the bath things got really freaky when my rounded tummy momentarily went up into a tentlike shape with a point. At any moment I thought Sigourney Weaver might appear in a onesie.

To add to the glamour of my relationship, apparently I am snoring like a demented tractor every night.

I have a marvelously glamorous moment in a restaurant debriefing the boss about Fashion Week. As I squeeze between tables on the way to the bathroom, I attempt to keep my bump off a nearby table and instead sweep my ass along the table behind me in a majestic arc, taking the two menus and a good bit of the tablecloth with me. Talk about dignity.

info

third-trimester hassles

These three complaints can start earlier, but they usually bug pregnant women the most in the last three months.

heartburn

What is it? Heartburn is that burning sensation you feel behind the breastbone, sometimes accompanied by the taste of small amounts of regurgitated food and stomach acid. It doesn't affect the baby.

Why does it happen? Because of the high levels of progesterone during pregnancy, which relaxes muscles, the muscular valve between the stomach and the esophagus (the tube connecting stomach and mouth) relaxes, and so stomach acid flows up into the esophagus and sometimes the mouth. It doesn't help that later in the pregnancy your uterus is encroaching on your tummy and squeezing it upward.

What can you do?

⑥ Eat several small meals slowly, rather than wolfing three main ones. Try to stay upright (sitting or standing) for 30 minutes after eating.

⑥ Avoid spicy, highly seasoned, fried, or fatty foods, chocolate, coffee, alcohol, carbonated drinks, spearmint, and peppermint, and anything with lots of chemical additives.

⑥ Wear loose clothing around your tummy.

⑥ Don't fold yourself up on the couch, because that squashes your tummy, and bend from the knees, not the waist, to pick things up.

⑥ If the heartburn is worse when you lie flat, try elevating your head by at least 6 inches with pillows, which will help to stop the yukky stuff flowing up into your mouth.

⑥ Try not to put on too much extra weight.

⑥ Don't smoke.

⑥ Try foods such as milk or yogurt that help to neutralize the stomach acid.

⑥ If none of this helps, ask your doctor to recommend an antacid that is suitable for use during pregnancy. (Avoid preparations containing sodium or sodium bicarbonate.)

backache

Why does it happen? Progesterone and relaxin relax the ligaments and joints of the spine and around the pelvis. This gets everything ready for childbirth but makes it hard to have good posture, especially when the weight of the baby puts pressure on your lower back and weakened tummy muscles and pulls the spine forward.

Lower back and leg pain can be caused by the pressure of the enlarging uterus on the sciatic nerve. The pain may pass as the baby's position changes. If it is very severe, you should tell your doctor. Sometimes working with a physical therapist can help.

What can you do?

⑥ Avoid standing and sitting for long periods of time. When you are standing, tilt your pelvis forward so that your butt tucks under, and keep your shoulders back; when sitting, get yourself well back into the seat, and put your legs up on another chair if possible.

⑥ Do some gentle stretching exercises recommended by your obstetrician or yoga teacher experienced in pregnancy.

⑥ The flatter your shoes, with good support, the better. This is no time for sparkly, aqua-go-green, platform thigh boots. Sadly.

⑥ Avoid twisting movements.

⑥ Bend from the knees when lifting things.

⑥ Avoid gaining too much weight—hate that one.

For backache itself

⑥ Have a massage.

⑥ Relax in a warm (not hot) bath or aim the shower spray at the painful area.

⑥ Apply a warm (not hot) hot-water bottle or heat pack.

⑥ If the pain is severe, ask your doctor to prescribe an analgesic safe for use during pregnancy.

⑥ If the pain is particularly bad, ask your doctor to refer you to a fully qualified, experienced trainer, osteopath, or chiropractor specializing in backache during pregnancy.

swelling and fluid retention

What is it? Swelling, most noticeably of the fingers, legs, ankles, and feet, also called edema, occurs because the body retains more fluid during pregnancy. (Your face can also swell, due to the effects of natural estrogen and cortisol, a steroid hormone, changing the distribution of fat in the body.)

Some fluid retention and swelling is perfectly normal and should cause no more than mild discomfort. However, if you feel that you are excessively puffy or if the edema persists for more than 24 hours at a time, you should inform your obstetrician. This can be normal, but it may be an early sign of preeclampsia (pregnancy-induced high blood pressure; see info in Week 31).

Why does it happen?   Hormonal changes can prompt the kidneys to hang onto salt, leading to fluid retention. There is much more fluid in your body in order to maintain the level of amniotic fluid and increase the water level in your blood to help the kidneys to get rid of waste.

Hot weather, standing, or sitting for long periods of time and high blood pressure are the most common causes of mild edema. It also occurs more commonly later in the day, as fluid pools in the ankles and feet—that's gravity for you. In the mornings you might see more puffiness in your eyelids and jawline. It is more likely if you're carrying a multiple pregnancy or excess weight.

What can you do?

⊚ Sit down and elevate your legs higher than 90 degrees or, preferably, lie down—on your left side, or on your back supported by a cushion so that your back is tilted 10 degrees or more.

⊚ Wear comfortable shoes.

⊚ Avoid socks or stockings with elasticized tops.

⊚ If the edema really bothers you, check out the range of support pantyhose (available in pregnancy sizes with extra tummy room)—and remember to put these on in the morning, when the swelling is less.

⊚ Don't add salt to any food. Avoid potato chips and other very salty foods.

⊚ Drink plenty of water to flush the body of waste products. Drinking extra water won't increase fluid retention—it may even reduce it.

⊚ If your fingers swell, remember to take off any rings before they become uncomfortably tight. (Some women wear any rings on a chain as a necklace.)

more possible tests

gestational diabetes

A temporary form of diabetes: the body does not produce enough insulin to keep pace with the increased blood sugar caused by pregnancy. (Some pregnancy hormones act against insulin.) It's routinely screened, usually by a blood test, between 24 and 28 weeks.

group B streptococcus (GBS)

You should be offered a test for this bacteria. Babies become really sick if they travel to the outside world down a vagina with GBS in it. A vaginal swab is usually routine in the third trimester, and if GBS is found you'll be prescribed antibiotics during the labor to clear it up. About 40 percent of women carry this bacteria in their vagina.

anemia

Your blood sample might also be checked for hemoglobin levels (indicating anemia—not enough iron).

Rh incompatibility

If your blood type is Rh⁻ and the baby's father's blood type is Rh⁺, your antibodies need to be checked.

↑sky

← baby

↙ ↓feet

your record

Have you had:	What have you done to treat it?
Heartburn?	
Backache?	
Fluid retention?	

WEEK

Nesting

Average approximate baby length this week from head to butt

in 1 2 3 4 5

what's going on

It's really hard to find a comfy position to sleep in. You'll find that pregnancy books often say not to lie on your back or your right side because this can lead to less blood flowing through the placenta, though in most pregnancies this isn't a problem. In any case, leaning against a pillow will solve it because to relieve the compression you only need to be tilted off your back by 10 degrees; lying on your side is unlikely to be a worry, but check with your doctor if you're concerned. Otherwise, you could nail a bucket to the floor, stick your head in it, and point the rest of your body toward the ceiling.

The baby is looking very babyesque at this point—plumper and rounder. The newborn-baby breathing rhythm is developing steadily; it's more regular, with fewer stops and starts. Weight: about 2 1/2 pounds.

7   8   9   10   11

DiARY

I think I've got interior design nesting rather than cleaning nesting. (Typical. Even when I'm nesting I don't want to do the dishes, I'd rather arrange some vases fairly artfully in the hallway. Tremendously useful skill around the house.) I am putting things in boxes and hiring large young men to come to the house while Matt is at work to move furniture from room to room.

Maybe it's not just about making a nest, but about throwing out stuff from the past, stuff you don't need, and working out what you do want. That sounds a bit deep. Luckily I'm so scatterbrained my mind, having thought, immediately moves on . . . to . . . Not. Thinking. Or . . . what?

Random thoughts

Must find out whether the religious hospital I'm going into will have full facilities on their day of worship if I happen to have a day of screaming. The idea of less than full catering and no obstetrician does not appeal.

Glamour check: I have discovered that pregnancy makes you sweat more—it's Mrs. Fluid has come to visit. If you're not retaining it, you're leaking it—or sometimes both at once. Not to mention all that extra blood in there. I tried a strong antiperspirant, but it only blocked my pores and I felt like I was carrying a marble around in my armpit for a couple of days. I had to go without any and then went back to deodorant. I can remember at 16 weeks when I skipped ahead in the books and thought, "God, look at 28 weeks." It seemed so far away. But now I'm here, in a flash. Better take some photos while I'm looking pregnant.

Peeing a zillion times a night. Trying to remember to do pelvic-floor exercises. Too boring for words.

My walking shoes smell disgusting. I have sprayed them with a French perfume called Fracas.

Childbirth classes start this week. I don't want to go. For some reason it feels like having to go to Sunday School. I can't stand those things where a Lorraine at the front of the classroom asks us all to share our feelings. I've already done the exercise classes, dammit. If I wanted to share my feelings with strangers I'd rent a billboard. I don't want to bond with the group. They're not going to be there when I have the child, or when it grows up. I don't care what they think or what they do, really. Perhaps I should just wear a name tag saying, "Hi! I'm a Churlish Bitch."

Our first childbirth class goes like this: a young, blonde Lorraine in a cuddly blue cashmere sweater and black leggings gives us all a sticky-label name tag as we walk in the door. We have to interview another couple (everyone is in a couple!—what's the world coming to?), and then introduce them to the class. "Garry and Dianne are drug dealers. They conceived accidentally during a police raid and their obstetrician is Dr. Feldman. Dianne intends to take at least a year off." Unfortunately it's not quite that interesting.

We are divided into men's and women's groups. I put my middle name on the name tag out of perversity so Matt has to keep squinting at my chest and saying things like, "Um . . . Mildred here is going out to work and I'm staying home." I feel it would be more entertaining if he could just admit he's forgotten the name of the mother of his child. Anyway, each group is asked to come up with a list of questions they would like the class to answer.

WOMEN

Can we eat during labor? (Yes, a bit in the early stages.)

Can we videotape the birth? (Depends on your doctor. Some would wear a party hat if you asked nicely. Some don't because it could be used in court against them.)

Will the hospital run as normal on the religious day of worship? (Yes.)

I want hints to help me in labor. (We'll be covering that.)

When is it really labor? (That too.)

Tell us every single pain relief option. (Certainly.)

What about if it's an emergency this small hospital can't deal with? (We have facilities for a sick mother. A sick baby will be sent to a larger hospital by ambulance. We can look after the baby adequately until the ambulance arrives.)

Is there a modem link in the delivery suite? Because I'd like my overseas relatives to see the birth on the Internet. (That's a very weird question, but I'm too polite to say so.)

Can I have twenty-seven people in the room when I'm giving birth? (No. You're a fruitcake.)

Do men ever display the nesting instinct? (Frankly, no.)

MEN

How do we know when it starts? (We'll be covering this.)

What should we expect on the day? (Ditto.)

How can we prepare? (Ditto.)

What support can we give? (All this will be revealed.)

Do WE get any drugs? (Good one, Matt.)

What is the man's role during labor? (Do whatever she tells you and be quick about it.)

What if we faint? (Keep up your meals and drinks during labor and sit down if you think you might faint.)

How to recognize signs of postpartum depression? (That will be discussed.)

What to bring and wear? (Ball gown.)

What to have ready at home? (Alcohol.)

What if the baby comes early and quickly? (Call the ambulance and follow their instructions.)

Young Lorraine, who is actually a Melissa, explains that the first lesson will be on signs that labor isn't far off (maybe hours or days). Signs include the "show," which is the mucus plug coming

out (she says that it might be the size of a dollar coin on your
undies, and possibly bloody and mucusy); and the "waters
breaking," which is about a cup of amniotic fluid leaking or
gushing out when the membranes break (she says don't get it on
the car upholstery because it rots it, so from 35 weeks I'll be
sitting on a tarp and four towels in the passenger seat of Matt's
precious van). I ask if it's true the waters smell of pickles. Melissa
looks sideways and lets us know it's a sweet smell that's actually,
ahem, like semen.

Other signs that labor may begin soon are: tummy dropping
as the baby's head engages with the pelvis, nesting and cleaning,
more pre-labor contractions, increased vaginal secretions, pelvic
pressure and heaviness in the groin.

Then Melissa points to a chart and explains the following parts
of a pregnant woman's anatomy: the vagina ("If you didn't know
where that was, you wouldn't be here"), cervix (the bit between
the vagina and the uterus), fetus, and fundus (the top of the
uterus). She explains that labor contractions begin in the fundus
and the pain radiates down to period-cramp territory in the lower
abdomen. Our bags should be packed by 35 weeks, as 37 weeks is
considered full term.

Two hours of this and I'm ready for a whiskey. Ready, willing,
but not able.

info

what are the signs of premature labor?

Even if you're feeling like pregnancy has gone on quite long enough, premature labor might be a bit of a freak-out as well. Always remember you're living in a developed country with large hospitals. (If you're living near a major metropolitan center, you should have the best available medical care for preemie babies; if you're in a rural or remote area, that access may not be the same.)

Labor is considered premature if it begins earlier than the thirty-seventh week of pregnancy. Signs that you may be in early labor are:

◉ cramps, like period pains, that may be accompanied by nausea, diarrhea, or indigestion.

◉ increasing pain or feeling of pressure in the lower back.

◉ unusual or persistent achiness or feeling of pressure in the pelvic floor, thighs, or groin.

◉ a watery or pinkish or brownish discharge, possibly preceded by the passage of the thick mucus plug (euwwwwww!) that has been blocking your cervix.

⑥ fluid from your vagina (your "waters breaking"), which means the amniotic sac has ruptured and some amniotic fluid is rushing or trickling out.

late bleeding

Any light bleeding or spotting in the second and third trimesters should be checked out immediately by your obstetrician to be absolutely sure. Two uncommon conditions that cause bleeding late in pregnancy are placenta previa and placental abruption.

placenta previa

With placenta previa, the placenta is attached to the lower part of the uterine wall, instead of the upper part, partially or completely blocking the way out. The risk of having placenta previa is increased if you have uterine scarring from previous cesarean sections or uterine surgery, you smoke, or there's more than one baby in there. If the bleeding is severe you may need an emergency cesarean.

placental abruption (abruptio placentae) or placental separation

Placental abruption is when the placenta comes away from the uterine wall too early. The amount of bleeding and also the amount of pain depend on how much of the placenta has come away. The cause is unknown, but it tends to be more common in women with elevated blood pressure and smokers. Sometimes the problem resolves itself and the pregnancy continues as normal. Sometimes the birth must be induced; in serious, sudden cases a cesarean is necessary.

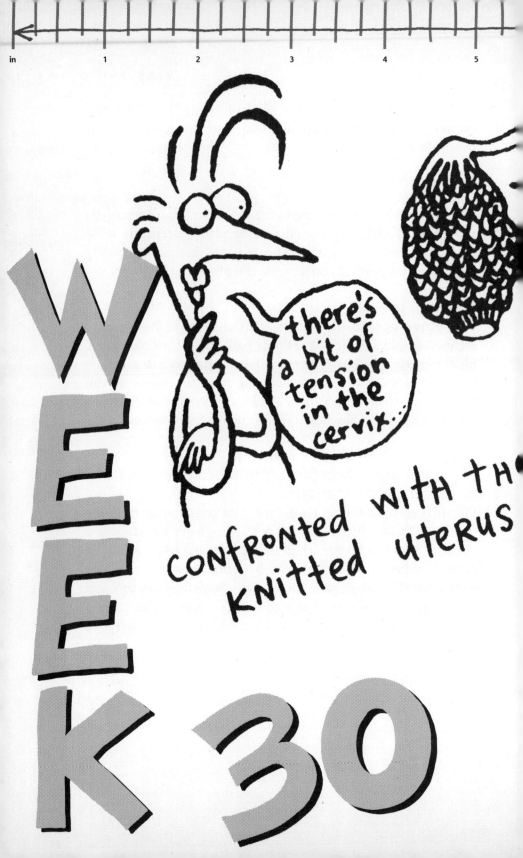

what's going on

Your breasts are STILL getting bigger. Will they ever stop? Yes. You might be feeling occasional pre-labor uterine contractions now, although most people don't feel them until the last weeks. Proper labor contractions last for 1 minute each, come at intervals of 5 minutes or less, gradually increase in intensity, and go on for at least an hour, and then after a while a baby comes out. So if that happens, you're probably really in labor.

This week and the following 3, the baby puts on fat at a greater rate. The skin is still a bit wrinkled, so there's room for the new fat underneath. The lanugo will start to fall out, although a full head of hair may stay. The eyes are fully open, but it can't be very interesting just watching all that hair floating around. Baby hiccuping starts to get more violent: you can feel the little jerks. Weight: about 3 pounds.

Diary — Thank God I go to see Marg's baby, Gloria. It reminds me that there's a reward at the end of all this. Marg's full of advice about the changing table arrangement, the best diaper covers, the best undershirts, etc. I must start taking notes.

Also go to see Dr. Herb.

He takes one look at me and says, "It must be soon."

"Soon!" I shriek. "It's 10 weeks away. I can't even begin to tell you what I have to get done before it arrives!"

There was a woman in the waiting room who'd come to give him a present. She had a 3-year-old with a narrow little face—this was the smallest and earliest surviving baby Herb had ever delivered. She came at 23 weeks and spent months in an incubator. Her mom was obviously madly in love with her little girl.

When Herb examines me, he smiles and says, "Your baby is big and healthy. It's going to be the opposite of that one you saw in the waiting room."

I hope this doesn't mean it's coming out at 57 weeks.

Herb agrees I have put on a lot of weight, but says, "Worry about it after the baby is born. Just don't eat junk food."

All the skinny girls at work put on more than 40 pounds during their pregnancies and lost it again afterward. You can't go on a weight-loss diet during pregnancy. You (well, all right then, I) can stop eating a Haagen Dazs a day though, which might help. I tell myself that it would be more dangerous for a baby if I didn't put on enough weight during pregnancy than if I ended up looking like a pivotal protagonist in *Moby Dick: The Miniseries*.

For a fashion designer, I've got nothing to wear. But how selfish, I think. I'd better shop for the baby. (Besides which, shopping is no fun anymore because after you've been walking for 15 minutes your feet feel like someone's been whacking them rhythmically with a baton for an hour.) I go to a posh shop and accidentally spend $277 on baby things like blankets and undershirts—honestly I didn't buy anything expensive at all. I become quite stupidly emotional over a tiny pair of socks for a newborn baby and start crying. Good God. (Let's face it, I'm liable to burst into tears during a tampon ad.)

Matt is being a prince—well, a prince's servant—still doing all the dishes and cooking most nights. (He tends to cut things up into infinitesimally small pieces, but never look a gift dinner in the mixed metaphorical mouth, I say.)

Hired the removalists again to move more furniture around. Getting there. This weekend had better go and look for a changing table, and that crib Uncle Stan said he'd pay for. More shelves being delivered. Matt just stands back and lets it all happen, and occasionally he shakes his head and mutters like one of the witches in *Macbeth*. At least I think he said "bubble."

Second week of childbirth classes. And tonight our special project is: Normal Labor. Melissa is slightly less perky. Perhaps she's been delivering babies for 36 hours.

Melissa gives us the old line about having faith in your body and the pain being part of a natural process. I can't help it, it sounds like a crock. While I have always thought childbirth was actually a design fault, it is strangely comforting to know that millions of women have done it.

What Melissa says is that the average for a first-time labor is 12–16 hours. The time is counted from the start of getting regular contractions. (Statistically, second and subsequent babies slither out after about 6 hours.) I'm still not clear about this 12–16 hours. It's roughly made up of 10–12 hours waiting for the cervix to dilate to 10 centimeters (first stage), and then say 2 hours pushing and shouting at people (second stage), as far as I can ascertain. After that there is a third stage of labor, when the placenta comes out, which nobody seems particularly interested in. If an injection of pitocin is given this takes between 10 and 30 minutes. If it comes out naturally, it's usually under an hour.

Next Melissa produces from her handbag a very startling pink knitted uterus with a cream cuff on it, which represents the cervix. I don't know where she got the pattern. She says your waters can break at any time before or during the labor, even right at the very end. At first the contractions last for 20 seconds, like a period cramp. They increase from 20 minutes apart to 5 minutes apart. During the last bit of the first stage, the contractions are longer and very intense and 3–5 minutes apart.

The second stage of labor is heralded by the "transition"—when the cervix is almost completely dilated (about 10 centimeters): wide enough for the baby's head to fit through. Ow. Ow ow OW. The contractions are only 1–3 minutes apart and last for up to 90 seconds. This is usually the stage when women scream for an epidural and are often refused.

"If you're abusive we know you're nearly there," says Melissa.

This sounds like a horrible stage when you can be shaky and vomit from the shock and stress, and you flake out for those tiny minutes between contractions.

At this point most of the men in the class move closer to their partners and take their hands. (You can tell they're thinking, "Oh you poor dear," and then, "Glad I don't have to do that bit.") They will not be so free with their fingers during the real thing: support people are advised that only two fingers be gripped by the laboring woman as any more fingers are easier to squish together, and even break. Support people are also advised to eat and drink and take rests.

After this stage, as far as I can see, a soft-toy baby comes out of a knitted uterus into a stuffed pelvis. Melissa advises us not to be too energetic in the early stages of labor before going to hospital as we'll need our strength later.

Apparently the very end of labor feels exactly like the urge to poo. Some women keep changing positions; some have their baby on all fours or a birth stool, or sitting up on the bed. Squatting is not something we do a lot of, so unless you're on one of those giant inflatable birth balls they have in some labor rooms it will probably be too much for your leg muscles.

This week was probably the perfect week to consider some of the mechanics of childbirth as I am just changing from major denial (well yes, I know I'm pregnant, but I don't think I actually want to go through childbirth) to major denial (look, I know I'm pregnant, but I really don't want to think about how this baby everyone keeps saying is so HUGE is going to get out—I feel like I'm going to give birth to a small apartment block).

Melissa says we can massage the perineum (the area in front of your anus) for several weeks before the birth, because it might make it less likely that the perineum skin tears during the last stage of childbirth. Sounds like an excuse for dusting off the vibrator to me. (Dr. Herb's view is it's a complete waste of time.) (The massage, not the vibrator.)

"Often we ask the dad if he wants to cut the cord," Melissa says. For some reason every woman in the class breaks up laughing. "Once the head is through, that's the hard bit done—unless you've got a really big baby and then the shoulders can be difficult." Oh dear.

Melissa then talks about the third stage of labor, which involves the expulsion of a large stuffed red stocking, with a veil around the edge that makes it look like a giant jellyfish, and a twisty gray cord hanging from it, which is the placenta and umbilical cord. At this point Melissa admits that somewhere she has a knitted breast as well. I hate to think what her tea cozies look like.

Then we watch two videos. The first one is narrated by a serious guy who says things like "some of the joy and happiness brought about by this happy event" and "this stained mucus plug" as if he were reading the Channel 4 news. This happy event and the stained mucus plug are both brought to us by somebody called Julie, who wears a yellow sweater until the second stage of labor, when she changes into a mauve silk negligee (bad move, really). At the hospital Julie wanders the corridors like Lady Macbeth and then ends up panting, which Melissa has said is not good so early in the labor. An obstetrician turns up in a hideous patterned sweater and holds one of Julie's legs while Scott, her husband, holds the other. Being in labor is probably the only time a woman wouldn't even notice this happening. Then the midwife squirts some cold detergent on Julie's private parts, which Melissa says is shocking behavior as it gives Julie quite a fright. "We like to give you a quick, warm wash," she says. The whole video is 15 minutes long, which I think is a little misleading.

The midwife holds the baby back so it doesn't come out in too much of a rush and tear Julie, and then the head comes out a very gray-blue and turns slowly before the rest slips out. By about this stage nearly every man in the room has gone into shock and half of them have tried to crawl into their partner's lap—forgetting that, with a 7-month pregnant woman, lap space is at a premium.

We watch a second video, starring a more hippie couple. (Why is it that in every picture, drawing, and video to do with pregnancy and childbirth the husband has facial hair?) Anyway, this woman gives birth on all fours and then scoops the baby up as if she does it every day.

Neither woman needs stitches. As if.

Back at home poor old Matt is squished into an area of the bed that's the size of an envelope. I waddle to the bathroom about six times a night and have taken to having under-desk naps at work.

And the mood swings! Matt never knows whether he's coming home to Medusa or Mrs. Cleaver.

One of the male models looks at me in the elevator at work and blurts out, "What happens to all that stomach . . . afterward?"

"I'm giving it to the Salvation Army," I reply.

info

premature birth

why does it happen?
About half the time, medical people don't know. Here are some possibilities:

⑥ over-distended uterus caused by more than one baby, or too much amniotic fluid.

⑥ incompetent cervix (incompetent my foot—what a RUDE medical term; it just means that your cervix isn't staying tightly closed enough).

⑥ early rupture of the membranes of the amniotic sac (waters breaking).

⑥ something wrong with the baby or the placenta.

⑥ the baby has died while still in the uterus (this is rare).

⑥ the mother has a disease, is underfed, or experiences a trauma (such as a car accident).

⊚ the mother's and father's blood types don't mix (rhesus incompatibility).

⊚ pregnancy in a diabetic woman.

⊚ the mom is a young teenager.

how early is too early?

Any baby born before 37 weeks is usually considered premature, or preterm. With specialist care, babies as young as 24 weeks can survive. By 30 weeks, there is a 90 percent survival rate, and more than 80 percent of these babies will be fine after a bit of special care. If there is enough warning, mothers are often given steroids to improve their baby's lung development.

special care

⊚ Most doctors try for a vaginal delivery if all seems well.

⊚ A pediatrician or neonatologist will be part of the medical team at any premature birth.

⊚ If your baby needs help with temperature regulation or breathing, it will be placed in an incubator or ventilator perhaps under a warming light, and taken to the hospital's intensive neonatal care unit.

⊚ Your baby's condition will be assessed using a test of responses at 1 minute and again at 5 minutes after birth, called the APGAR test.

⊚ If the lungs are not developed enough, your baby will be given surfactant-replacement therapy, which uses an artificial protein in place of surfactant, a substance that normally completely coats the lungs in the last weeks of pregnancy to prevent them collapsing.

⊚ If your baby can't breastfeed right away, the doctors may have you pump your milk and feed it to the baby through a feeding tube. If for any reason your baby can't take your breast milk, they can be fed formula through a special tube.

⑨ Premature babies grow and thrive better if exposed to massage, skin-to-skin contact with parents or caregivers, soft music, recordings of heartbeats or the mother's voice, and water beds or hammocks that simulate movement in the uterus.

common preemie characteristics

Premature babies differ from full-term babies in a number of usually temporary ways.

⑨ Obviously, premature babies weigh less than full-termers.

⑨ They are small, red, wrinkly, and frail, with relatively large head and hands.

⑨ Their skin is pale, and blood vessels can easily be seen underneath because there is not much fat.

⑨ There is a layer of fine hair (lanugo) on the body.

⑨ Their motor functions, including breathing and feeding, are less efficient and their cry is not as lusty as that of a full-term newborn baby.

⑨ They tend to be less expressive than full-termers—they sleep most of the time, and when they are awake they do not make much eye contact or respond to people talking to or touching them. They also tend to be irritable. Can't blame them really.

 See Premature Babies in Help.

your record

What experiences have you had of childbirth?
Have you been to a birth? What was it like?

What videos and descriptions have impressed you
either positively or negatively?

what's going on

Hello stretch marks here, there, and possibly everywhere! What a splendid mauve, perhaps an attractive eggplant color, or is it hot pink? Pay attention to your posture, as your tummy will be putting you off balance.

The baby can blink or close its eyes when a bright light is shone onto your tummy. There's a lot of brain action going on: receiving and sending lots of signals through the nervous system, maybe testing out the idea of thinking, possibly wondering how long it has to hang out in a hairy swamp. The baby has definite awake and sleeping times and are still usually roughly the opposite of yours. Weight: about 3 1/3 pounds.

Average approximate baby length this week from head to butt

in   1   2   3   4   5

Guard against madness —
DON'T IRON YOUR UNDiES!

DiARY I'm a little breathless because my lungs are all squished up. Unfortunately this does not make me sound like Marilyn Monroe singing "Happy Birthday, Mr President"; it's more like an over-exerted warthog. Also, I have a constant ache where the ligaments from the baby area extend down to the groin. Leg cramps keep waking me up at night at 4 A.M., and I can't get back to sleep.

Beck says it's probably not magnesium deficiency but a circulation problem and maybe I should walk shorter distances every day instead of 1 1/2 miles every other day. Maybe I get worse cramps during the nights when I don't walk.

During my walk today a huge truck pulled up at the park with rolls of wire in the back, and a big burly guy in a reflective vest and cutoffs got down from the cab, walked around to the passenger seat, and collected a 2-year-old girl with a pageboy haircut.

"Come on, darling," he said. And they went to feed the seagulls.

It made me think that having children brings out the best kindness and the worst temper in us. And I hope it will bring out the best in me, not the worst. Or at least when it brings out the worst there will be someone else to take up the slack while I go and bite some telephone poles.

Matt and I spend an afternoon looking at cribs. It's amazing—some of them even LOOK dangerous, having gaps that a rhinoceros could practically climb out of. Not much more to buy now, but it would be nice if the washer-dryer fairy paid a visit.

Never speak too soon about household appliances. Just after I write that bit I notice that the enamel is flaking off the toaster onto our toast, so no doubt I've been ingesting bits of plutonium or aluminum or something.

Then this creepy guy turns up to service the heater, which I thought should have a new fan because the old one sounded a bit like the Concorde landing. He opens up the front and says, "It's a wonder you're not dead."

"Pardon?"

"This thing's been leaking carbon monoxide. You could have nodded off to sleep on the couch and never woken up. I'm surprised you're still alive."

Well.

Finally manage to take action and walk out the front door, burst into tears and call Matt, only to get his voice mail. Damn, damn, damn, he is probably in the back alley of the shop explaining succulents to some dopey businessman who thinks hydroponics is a grunge band, so I call the poison control hotline, who put me onto a local hospital where FINALLY, just before I think I'll go mad, a woman in the drug information department explains that unless I have experienced the symptoms of carbon monoxide poisoning (severe nausea, severe headaches, and severe lethargy and faintness) nothing will have crossed the placenta, and even if it has the likely result will have been a lack of oxygen getting to the baby, similar to what would happen if I smoked or walked around in the traffic all day, in which case the baby might be a little small.

"No," I assure her. "The general consensus is that I am having a baby approximately the size of Danny deVito."

"Well," she says, "nothing to worry about then."

Phew.

It is really very uncomfortable now. Beck has prescribed a grab bag of different supplements for me (which she hates doing) to try to bring down my fluid retention. Vitamin E, vitamin C, dandelion-leaf tincture (all at very precisely calibrated doses or it won't work), a complicated custom herbal mixture that tastes like a gasoline by-product with bats' ears in it, and I'm sure if she thought it would help I would have to hang upside down every 3 hours as well. Dr. Herb just shrugs his shoulders and says he hopes it helps because he can't give me drugs.

Every now and then I forget I'm pregnant for a minute or two, and then the baby kicks or I have to move or something and remember. Matt is being very sympathetic. I can't believe I have put on 37 pounds. From behind I look like two driver's-side airbags going off.

Go and buy some 100-percent cotton crib sheets—very hard to find. Another pregnant woman and I both put a hand on the last set. We look at each other.

She says graciously, "You take it, you're more pregnant than me."

Sisterhood!

"Most people," says a Lorraine-like sales assistant, "don't buy 100-percent cotton because they have to iron the sheets."

"Iron the sheets?!" I shriek. "Are they mad?!"

Our third childbirth class: when to come to the hospital. Melissa says to come to hospital when your contractions are 5 minutes apart, the waters have broken, you have any bleeding, or you're overwrought, but to call the hospital and your obstetrician first in case they've all stepped out for a daiquiri. No, to tell them what's been happening. Once you get to the hospital a nurse will inspect you before calling in your obstetrician.

Here are the main points I shall have to memorize.

False contractions are irregular, don't increase in intensity, and usually go away if you lie down.

The water breaking can be a tiny trickle or 1–2 liters of amniotic fluid coming out. Put on a pad. You're supposed to write down the time your water breaks and note the quality and color of the fluid. If there's a stain or blood in the water, tell your nurse or hospital staff immediately, by phone.

Don't call everyone and tell them you're in labor or they'll all be at the house or turning up at the hospital or getting times wrong and starting accidental rumors. Don't play hockey—conserve your energy for the labor.

Everyone is on the edge of their seat. This is what we came for—a bit of a chat about the real thing. Mind you, I thought there'd be a lot more beanbag action, and a lot more practice breathing. Apparently it's out of fashion. I am so glad Melissa is not the type to say, "Pinch your hand as hard as you can," each week to demonstrate the pain of labor. Because it's a bit like saying, "See that little dinghy? It's kind of like an aircraft carrier."

Melissa says not to worry if you poop during labor, and you probably won't because diarrhea is often an early sign of labor so you'll have gotten rid of it all before you deliver. Anyway, now that I've peed on my own floor because my pelvic-floor muscles are so hopeless, I suspect I can poop on the hospital bed, no problem.

Everyone is rather surprised to learn a few things. No wonder the baby comes out with its eyes closed—otherwise the first thing it would see is its mother's . . . ahem . . . asshole.

At that point I thought things would be pretty much all over but I'd forgotten there's the third stage—the placenta along with some blood and fluid comes out. (In order to demonstrate the placenta, Melissa drops the "baby" on the carpet, which she promises not to do if she's assisting at any of our births.) And then the obstetrician will do a bit of classy embroidery on any tears or cuts. Melissa gives us the hospital's March stats: forty-five deliveries, twenty-two intact perineums. Yikes.

info

preeclampsia

what is it?

It used to be called preeclamptic toxemia (if your mom had it, that's what it would have been called). It only ever happens in pregnancy, and it's diagnosed if your blood pressure is 140/90 or higher and you have extra protein in your urine. Symptoms might include facial swelling, headaches that don't resolve with pain medication, visual disturbances, or abdominal pain. If you have any of the symptoms, tell your doctor.

Preeclampsia is a serious condition that affects up to 7 percent of pregnant women, usually in the second half of preg-nancy. Occasionally the onset will coincide with labor and, rarely, it can occur after delivery. The cause has still not been established.

Preeclampsia can interfere with the placenta, stunting the baby's growth and depriving it of oxygen. It can cause the baby to come early and damage the mother's kidneys, nervous system, and blood vessels.

Sometimes preeclampsia can get worse really quickly: symptoms (apart from fluid retention) may include persistent headache, blurred vision, seeing flashing lights, upper or mid-abdominal pain, irritability, nausea, and vomiting. Women being treated for preeclampsia, if not hospitalized, should get emergency medical treatment at the onset of any of these symptoms.

Severe preeclampsia can escalate into eclampsia, which is a life-threatening condition for mother and fetus but is now extremely rare because of better medical monitoring. Eclampsia can cause convulsions, kidney failure, and coma. Blood vessels in the uterus go into spasm and cut down the blood supply to the baby.

check ups

Early detection and treatment mean preeclampsia is better managed. Your urine sample and blood pressure are checked at each prenatal visit to the obstetrician or prenatal clinic in the third trimester, and you should tell your pregnancy caregiver about any puffiness or swelling. (Having only one of the preeclampsia symptoms, such as fluid retention, doesn't mean you have preeclampsia.)

You're more likely to get preeclampsia if you had high blood pressure before you were pregnant; have a family history of preeclampsia or high blood pressure; had or have kidney disease; have diabetes; have had or are having a multiple pregnancy; had preeclampsia in a previous pregnancy; are a teenager or an older mom; or the pregnancy is your first.

sample

café latté to go

DO NOT GET 'EM CONFUSED

treatment

There is no conclusive evidence, but many people believe that good levels of calcium in your diet can reduce the risk of preeclampsia. Treatment for mild preeclampsia may include bed rest at home or in a hospital, and careful monitoring of you and your baby. Tests may include blood and urine checks, monitoring of the fetal heart rate, and ultra-sounds.

If the condition progresses to severe preeclampsia or is advanced when diagnosed, you'll need to go to the hospital. You may need medication to wrestle your blood pressure into submission, and your labor may be induced, or you may have a cesarean, depending on whether you respond to treatment, the state of your uterus, and how advanced the pregnancy is.

WEEK 32

what's going on

Your lungs are getting stronger, although because of all the pressure you may feel breathless if you overdo it. You may be starting to get a bit sick of the whole pregnancy thing. It's uncomfortable being this big, you're running out of outfits, and as for sleeping well—ha!

The baby's lungs are stronger too, but not fully ready to go yet. The baby is filling out with fat, although it still looks a bit on the skinny side. It might be upside down in readiness for the lunge to the outside world. This is pretty much your complete baby item, covered in vernix. If the baby was born now it would open its eyes and take a peek at the world (except it can't focus on much at this age and would look endearingly cross-eyed). Weight: about 3 3/4 pounds.

in   1   2   3   4   5

Average approximate baby length this week from head to butt

DiARY

I walk into Dr. Herb's office.
"You look tired and bloated," he says.
Charmed, I'm sure.

He says the insomniac sore legs when lying down are probably due to the fluid retention. He listens to the baby's heartbeat, asks if the baby's moving (is it ever: the Blini loves to rhumba all night long), and measures the length of the uterus.

"The baby's doing beautifully—you're doing really well," he says.

It's very kind the way he does this sort of positive bit after he tells me I look like shit (in the nicest possible way).

There are no safe drugs for fluid retention during pregnancy, Herb explains.

"Why can't I take diuretics?" I whine.

"Two reasons. They reduce placental blood flow, and they can mask the symptoms of preeclampsia."

Oh, all right, smartypants.

He sends me around the corner to a pathology lab, where I get a blood test from a Lorraine to check if there's a high level of uric acid in the blood or my platelets are at all deranged—both signs that I might be susceptible to preeclampsia. I quite like the idea of my platelets being deranged. I'm so responsible these days there should be some part of me acting like an idiot, but on second thought I can definitely do without preeclampsia. I have to come again next week because I'm retaining so much fluid Herb wants to keep an eye on it.

Week 4 of the childbirth class: Melissa's Reader's Digest version of stuff that might happen that isn't your ideal plan. Forceps might be used if you're too tired to push any more, the baby seems to be staying put, you've been pushing for too long, or there are signs of fetal distress. Usually you'll get an epidural first. I can see why when Melissa holds up a pair of forceps. They look like very upmarket, Italian, oversized salad servers from one of those designer shops full of stuff that people don't really need but has Alessi written all over it. There are two types: rotator forceps (also known as Kiellands forceps) and lift-out forceps.

Then there's the rather sophisticated-sounding vacuum extractor, a suction cup that they can stick on the baby's head and, well, pull it out. (It's a vacuum in the sense of a plunger, not the type you do the carpet with.) Melissa sits there absentmindedly playing with the soft-toy baby on her lap. So far she's folded it in half and is waving one of its feet past its ear.

Emergency cesareans are performed when a large baby is stuck, the cervix just isn't getting any wider, or the baby is really distressed. Usually you'll get an epidural or a spinal block to numb the lower half of your body usually included in the epidural is a long-lasting morphone derivative. "Hi baby! Mommy's reeeeally stoned!" Typically you're on a drip for up to 24 hours and have a catheter for peeing for up to 24 hours. The baby feeds as normal, and the dad, another helper, or a staff member does the diaper changes and baths and stuff.

What about the bizarre-sounding induction or inducement (as in "He offered me an illegal inducement, Your Honor, and I booked him for aggravated bribery")? An obstetrician may bring on (induce) labor if you're more than 1–2 weeks overdue, if your little bub isn't growing well, or if you have preeclampsia. Melissa says she knows of a doctor who induced a baby because its mother didn't want a Scorpio, and a doctor who refused to induce a baby on the Fourth of July for some nutty patriots.

Then Melissa talks about stillbirth. Everyone in the room goes very quiet. She says she doesn't want to talk about it, but she has to because it does still happen rarely that a baby is born dead, or is born with so many problems that it slips away from life a few days later. She says that in the case of a stillbirth, the baby often hasn't moved for a day or two before the labor. So always call your obstetrician if you haven't felt the baby move for 12 hours— although usually the baby's fine and just quiet.

If a baby is stillborn, the hospital organizes to have photos taken and inked footprints on a card done, even if you don't want these mementos at the time. (One bereaved mom called after 3 years to get hers.) Melissa's eyes fill with tears as she talks, and so do mine.

info

birth plan

what is it?

You write down all the things you want to happen during your labor. It's not a legal contract, but rather a memo of understanding between you and your birth attendants. Some women create specific birth plans; other choose to "go with the flow." Whatever you decide to do, it's a good idea to discuss with your obstetrician or midwife about their usual procedure, about the policies of the hospital or birth center, and about things such as playing the music of your choice during labor, family and friends being able to visit soon after the birth, and so on. You may not be able to have your own way on everything—this is the time to find out.

Discuss your birth plan with your obstetrician or midwife early, so that you're not still negotiating as the baby's coming out. Give your doctor a copy of the plan and tuck a copy away in your handbag.

what's in it?

The following plan format is based on a best-case scenario, but what if there are unexpected difficulties (induced labor, forceps delivery, emergency cesarean)? For example, if you have a cesarean you will probably want to keep the baby with you for a bit, not have it whisked away immediately for weighing and measuring, as this time can be very important for bonding with your baby. You will need your obstetrician to agree, so it's good to have it in your birth plan.

Your plan may be a long and detailed list of what you want to happen at every stage of your labor, just a letter to your obstetrician or midwife saying what you want, or a bullet-point list of the stuff you think is most important. It might include:

ⓖ who will be there.

ⓖ what you'd like to have around you to help you feel more comfortable and relaxed, such as music, massage oils, and photos.

ⓖ what clothes you would like to wear during the birth (hats and gloves are passé, and don't forget that anything that goes lower than your hips is likely to come off very second best in the stain department).

ⓖ whether you want a tape recording, photos, or a video of the birth, and who will be taking these.

ⓖ how, and how often, you would like to be monitored—some fetal monitors inhibit walking around.

ⓖ whether you would like to be able to eat in the early stages and drink through the labor.

ⓖ whether you would like an IV during labor (a catheter in your vein which can be hooked up to fluids).

ⓖ whether you would have a catheter (a tube coming out of your urethra, which pee automatically flows from)—yes/no/only if you have an epidural and can't feel whether your bladder is full.

ⓖ at what point you would like to be offered pain relief.

◉ what your preferred pain relief options are.

◉ what delivery position you'd prefer—squatting, sitting, or on all fours perhaps.

◉ whether you object to an episiotomy (a cut made at the entrance to the vagina to preempt the tearing).

◉ whether you want to touch your baby's head as it crowns (peeps out for the first time).

◉ who gets to lift the baby up first—maybe the baby's father, or you, or the obstetrician or midwife?

◉ who you would like to cut the umbilical cord.

◉ whether you want to keep the baby with you until *you* decide the staff can weigh it.

◉ whether you would accept drugs to speed up the normal delivery of the placenta.

pain relief options

Way before you're due, the following people will give you advice on pain relief: your obstetrician, your midwife, your partner; plenty of people who haven't had a baby; plenty who have; and a large man named Trevor you meet at a leather bar.

The final decision rests with you. You can choose the pain relief you'd like for an ideal delivery, but accept that you may have to resort to, say, a cesarean. Having a backup plan means that you

HYPNOSIS: would you RespoNd well?

won't have to make any spur-of-the-moment decisions about pain relief during labor, if for example it lasts longer or is more painful than you ever expected.

non-drug methods

The following non-drug methods of pain relief are often suggested (for each of these, faith in the method will help—if you're skeptical now, you may be a lot more so when you're yelling):

◎ acupuncture.

◎ reflexology (a form of acupressure massage of the feet, hands, and ears).

◎ aromatherapy—this is *not* pain relief, it's just dickering with the atmosphere.

◎ breathing and meditation techniques—these need to be learned and practiced before labor.

◎ massage—this also needs to be practiced before labor by the person who will give it.

HeAto Pack

◎ moving around—keeping mobile can help take pressure off your back, as well as distract you from the pain; some women find that standing or squatting positions are much more comfortable during contractions and childbirth.

◎ hydrotherapy—a warm shower or bath will help to relax you; sitting in water can provide pain relief by supporting the abdominal wall and decreasing the pressure on muscles during contractions.

◎ localized heat—hot towels and heat packs can help mask pain and reduce muscle cramps and spasms.

◎ vocalization—groaning, chanting, or singing to "release" pain, otherwise known as Just. Plain. Yelling.

◎ transcutaneous electrical nerve stimulation (TENS)—a machine delivers a very low electric current to stimulate the skin through pads attached to either side of the spine, creating a tingling sensation. This current can block the pain signals coming from the uterus. This method only offers slight pain relief, but some women find it is enough, and it can be safely used throughout labor.

◎ hypnosis—if you respond well to hypnosis, you can reach a state of consciousness where you are aware of what is happening but don't perceive it as painful (but you would *really* want to have practiced this one).

◎ music (more dickering with the atmosphere, and be warned— a lot of people make elaborate birth tapes and end up throwing them across the labor room).

the hard stuff

Gas Gas, also known as inhalation analgesia, is nitrous oxide ("laughing gas") under various brand names, inhaled during contractions through a rubber mask. It is generally accepted that it eases the perception of pain but doesn't provide a complete block. Some women find that just the distraction of using the mask helps to take their mind off the pain. Others find the mask claustrophobic (a mouthpiece may be available). Gas can be used safely throughout labor and appears to have very little effect on the baby. It makes some people feel sick and light-headed.

Epidural and spinal block Many women request an epidural. First, a local anesthetic is injected into your back. Next, a fine, hollow needle is inserted between two vertebrae in your lower back, then a catheter is inserted via the needle, and anesthetic is injected into it. The catheter allows epidural drugs to be placed in the right spot in the back to block pain, and the continued administration of painkillers throughout labor and delivery. The anesthetic takes effect within a few minutes. The whole procedure usually takes about 30 minutes and must always be performed by an experienced anesthesiologist or nurse anethestist.

An epidural goes into the lower back tissue that surrounds the sac containing the spinal cord and spinal fluid, whereas a spinal block goes directly into the spinal fluid and so works quicker (it is often used in a cesarean delivery when speed is important).

Epidurals wear off after 1 or several hours depending on how much is used—they can be topped off during a long labor. A spinal block is a one-time injection that lasts 1–4 hours.

These are the only methods of pain relief currently available that take away all perception of pain yet allow you to stay conscious. That's why epidurals and spinal-block injections are used for cesareans.

An epidural or a spinal block for a cesarean is dosed differently than for labor. It numbs all sensation in the abdomen and also affects the nerves in the legs, making them feel very heavy, and nerves in the bladder (so you'll probably have a catheter inserted in your bladder because you won't know when you're peeing). Epidurals and spinals used to block pain in labor without numbing the legs and bladder are now routine in some hospitals.

Epidural anesthetic is often used when women are in great pain, if the baby is in an awkward position (such as breech), if it's a multiple birth, or with a forceps or vacuum delivery. An epidural can sometimes make it difficult for you to push because you can't feel the strong second-stage contractions. You can ask to have the concentration of the drug reduced or the rate of its administration slowed so that you can feel the contractions again.

There is very little risk involved with having an epidural or a spinal block administered. Occasionally an epidural only blocks pain in part of your abdomen, but the anesthesiologist can often fix that sometimes requiring the replacement of the epidural catheter. Less than 1 percent of women who have had an epidural report having a headache lasting up to a few days. Having an epidural or spinal block in itself won't affect your baby.

Narcotics Narcotics, usually given as injections or through an IV during the first stage of labor, dull the sensation of pain by stimulating opiate receptors in the brain and spinal cord.

The injection takes about 20 minutes to work and it lasts 1–3 hours. Side effects can include headache, blurred vision, mood changes, feeling well away with the fairies, and nausea. If given in large doses, it may make the baby sleepy and affect its breathing—

this is usually remedied by giving the baby a little oxygen or a drug after the birth to reverse the effects.

Local anesthesia The two most common forms of local anesthesia given during labor are a pudendal nerve block, which involves an injection to numb the lower vagina and perineum; and perineal anesthesia, injected into the perineum to reduce "discomfort" or, most commonly, to perform an episiotomy. Both types of anesthetic take effect within a few minutes. Minimum doses are used so as not to affect the baby.

General anesthetic This is almost never used during labor, but is sometimes necessary or preferred for cesareans, especially in an emergency. Except in special circumstances, an epidural or spinal block is safer and better for mother and baby during a cesarean.

more info on childbirth

All the pregnancy books listed in Week 2 have some birth info.

Find a childbirth education association in your city.

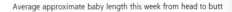

7   8   9   10   11

what's going on

You feel like there's not another thing that could be fitted inside you, not even a Mars Bar. Well, maybe a Mars Bar. Your navel is probably sticking out.

All the baby really needs now is more surfactant to coat its lungs and some more fat. It has an excellent chance of survival if it comes out now. As well as blinking, the baby is starting to learn to focus its eyes on close things like its own extremities and the umbilical cord. Weight: about 4 pounds.

WEEK 33

DiARY

I've been reading even more lists in books and hospital pamphlets about what to take to hospital: pillows, heat pad, and a birth ball; sanitary napkins the size of Manhattan; every beauty aid known to woman-kind, including "setting equipment" (one book apparently thinks you'll be giving yourself a home perm) and mascara for that touch-up during a difficult second stage of labor. PLUS: clothes for the baby, including booties (get out), bonnet (oh, shut up), undershirt, sleeper with legs (what?), and bunting with legs (stop it); cameras for still photos and videos (no thanks); change or a phone card to call people up ("Hello, I'd like to order a bunting. No, I don't know what it is"); books and magazines; your address book and notepaper to write thank-you letters for the flowers and presents (don't they know all you'll want to do is sleep?); and while you're about it, possibly some occasional furniture, a tuba, and, oh, maybe a kayak.

I've checked the hospital's policy on giving out info about the birth: luckily they refuse to tell anyone anything. Having confirmed her presence with the switchboard, the parents of my friend Fatimah drove straight to the hospital when she was in labor and tried to force their way into the delivery room while she was yelling at them to go away. Most unseemly. And I won't be leaving a message on the answering machine saying we've gone to the hospital. In fact I'm going to leave a message saying, "I haven't gone to the hospital, I'm just not answering the phone. Do not call the hospital. Repeat, and this means you, Aunt Peg, do not call the hospital. Leave a message."

Another fluid-retention vigilance visit to Dr. Herb to have blood pressure checked. The waiting room is an endless parade offering excellent people-watching opportunities. Today there is a very old man sitting in the corner sucking on his dentures so vigorously you can hear it coming down the corridor, and a couple who look straight out of the pages of Italian *Vogue*. Her: full, heavy makeup, hair done by the caring hands of a professional in the last 5 hours, Manolo Blahnik shoes, Armani suit, gold jewelry, and diamonds the size of small mammals. Him: full-length suede overcoat, tailored suit, silk tie, designer specs, carefully cultivated two-day growth. Not a hair out of place, not a piece of lint. I can't imagine what they would do with a baby. Put it in a vase, maybe.

I have plenty of time to look around—and to baby-sit a 6-week-old bundle whose mother is in with Dr. Herb. The Lovely Lorraine has gone off down the corridor to do something and has handed me a squirmy package who looks like she has nothing but disdain for the likes of my empty boozooms. Turns out she was halfway through a feeding when her mom finally got to go in. Dr. Herb is running about 2 hours late. Luckily I have taken some sketches and a report to work on.

When it's my turn, I climb up on the bed thing, which is so narrow it always reminds me of being on a ship (especially when I was feeling sick). Dr. Herb gets out his tape to measure the height of the uterus and feels my stomach and starts laughing.

"My, it's a whopper," he says.

Now, don't get me wrong. If I were on a fishing trip with somebody, or the boss was telling me about a pay raise, or an Italian sailor was taking off his pants in a sexual fantasy, the words "My, it's a whopper" could be exceedingly welcome. When the phrase refers, however, to something that has to come out of your vagina, sometimes referred to amusingly as the birth canal in a pathetic attempt to make it sound bigger, like, say, the Panama Canal, well, it is a different kettle of episiotomies entirely.

Dr. Herb's approach to the big-baby question is basically to wait and see what happens during labor. He says that ultrasounds have proven notoriously unreliable in judging whether a baby's head will fit through the middle of its mom's elvis. I mean pelvis. I suppose I had better read a bit more about cesareans, just in case. I have a mental picture of a whole lot of people with miners' helmets on, carrying coils of rope, peering up my vagina and shouting, "Come out, you great big thing!"

Dr. Herb also promises to refer me to a skin specialist who can remove the moles and skin tags that have gone berserk, but he says any mole or tag removal should wait until at least 3 months after the baby is born because they often disappear by themselves. (Not the babies, the moles.)

The fluid retention is really getting me down. I'm from a generation that has been taught (wrongly as it happens) that you can be somehow in control of your body—even change its essential shape by diet and exercise, or surgery. The feeling of being totally OUT of control—along for the ride, part of a biology experiment—is kinda disconcerting.

An uneasy feeling grows that the Crocodile Hunter is outside my house with a film crew, waiting to breathlessly narrate the next bit of my life. "G'day. Now the Madeline has only 6 weeks to go," he whispers to the camera, as he crouches behind the hibiscus. "Inside, she is groaning and puffing every time she lifts her enormous weight from the couch. She is now totally demented about getting the nursery set up, and if her mate, Matt, does not perform the act of cleaning his crap out of his room by the agreed deadline of 35 weeks, she will eat his head. Crikey."

Matt, fully apprised of the whopperiness of our offspring, has taken to calling it Gigantor instead of the Blini. I am running out of wry smiles.

My dreams are getting weirder and weirder. The night before last I dreamt that Matt left me and took the furniture, and I forgot to ask him if he was interested in seeing the baby after it was born. Then last night I dreamt I had given birth and then one of the nurses (who were all dressed in pastel French maids' uniforms— a very sartorially satisfactory dream) said, "There was another cord hanging out so we followed it back in, and it was attached to another baby, which has been hiding behind the uterus the whole time. So now you've got two."

Week 5 of childbirth classes: Melissa devotes the night to breastfeeding. I must admit I have kind of blanked out about breastfeeding. After Melissa wipes the floor with my illusions and severely bashes up my expectations, I fully realize that if I breastfeed I must accept that for several months I won't be able to (a) sleep, (b) work, (c) speak, (d) twirl tassels in opposite directions while they are attached to my nipples.

It's just that apparently you have to feed the little monsters at least every 4 hours in the early days, and apparently you're supposed to be awake while that happens. I can't imagine who designed this system. No wonder women in some other cultures aren't allowed to do any work or housework or even get out of bed for the first few weeks after childbirth.

And apparently for the full benefits that everyone raves about (boosting the baby's immune system, annoying old fuddy-duddies who simply go berserk at the sight of a publicly bared bosom, and so on), you need to breastfeed for a minimum of 6 months.

Melissa drops a few hints: go to the bathroom and wash your hands before you breastfeed, and have a set-up next to your chair with a glass of water, phone, and so forth on it. You see, I had imagined I could pop out of a long office meeting and whack the baby on a gland for, say, 7 minutes before handing it to a passerby and rushing back in. But apparently babies can stay on for up to half an hour each side! And sometimes they want it and sometimes they don't! And it might not be the 7 minutes you choose! And you can't just fill them up when it suits you because it takes 2–3 hours to "fill up" the breasts with milk again! Outrageous!

There are an awful lot of instructions about breastfeeding, but at least everyone now admits it can be really difficult. Plus Melissa is pretty sure that most of the midwives and lactation consultants (bet that looks good on a resume) at this hospital have their story straight, and we won't be plagued by seven different recommended methods while we're learning. Eventually ("they" say) you can pop a baby on your breast upside down in the dark while riding a horse backwards sidesaddle, but in the beginning it can be all rather laborious. Of course some people go at it as if they've been doing it forever.

When your breasts get engorged—have too much milk—they get really big and hard and painful, and that's when you get some chilled cabbage leaves out of the fridge and put one in each bra cup. Nobody really knows why it works, but I'd like to meet the person who worked it out.

The whole idea of expressing breast milk—pumping it out and putting it in bottles—which I'll have to do if I go back to work (or even leave the house without the baby at any point), seems damned weird. I can remember seeing rows and rows of dairy cows being milked and am starting to have visions of myself that are along the same lines.

We have reached the point with the fluid retention where the disgusting-tasting dandelion-leaf tincture I'm taking only goes so far toward keeping me distinguishable from a hot-air balloon. Now I just have to put up with it. Unless my blood pressure goes up as well, there's no danger to the baby. I can't find my Fat Boots. In the vague frame of mind I'm in, they'll probably turn up in the crisper. I specialize in sentences that are in search of an endi . . .

info

what to arrange before the hospital

◉ Go to prenatal classes, and do your reading. Labor and delivery are unpredictable, and it is very helpful if you and your partner or labor support person at least have *some vague idea* of what you might be in for.

◉ Write your birth plan if you decide to have one (see info in Week 32).

◉ Organize child care for your other child or children: this may need to be available at a moment's notice—even in the middle of the night—so it's a good idea to have a first choice and a backup. Make sure the kids are well briefed on the plan so they are not freaked out when they find you gone.

◉ Plan your transportation to the hospital; don't drive yourself. Avoid freeways if you can—they are hard to escape from when there's a traffic jam.

◉ Try to have nursery items and baby clothes collected by about now, just in case. Wash all baby clothes in a mild detergent before you'll need 'em.

◉ Have a freezer stocked full of easy food, ready for the first few weeks at home. You could prepare soups, pasta sauces, quiches, pies, lasagnes, or casseroles. Put it this way—you won't want to be plucking any chickens. When you go home your priorities will be (a) baby care, (b) sleep, and (c)—there is no c.

⑥ Have some light, nutritious early-labor food, such as home-made chicken stock, beef broth, or pureed fruit, in the freezer.

⑥ If you can afford it, arrange a house cleaner (friend, relative, or agency) for the first few weeks at home, especially if you know you're having a cesarean.

⑥ Order diaper wash service, if you plan to use it—or get a few packages of newborn-sized disposable diapers.

⑥ Install the baby seat in the car, and practice buckling and unbuckling with a teddy bear. You'll need it to take the baby home.

⑥ Find out what labor aids your hospital maternity ward or birth center can provide during labor and what you might need to bring in yourself—does it provide tape players for instance? Always double-check, when calling to say you're coming in, that whatever you need is still available just in case it's been booked by someone else.

⑥ When the time comes, phone your obstetrician or independent midwife and your hospital or birth center to tell them you're in labor and ask about when you should come in.

to take to the hospital

Your hospital or birth center may give you a list in advance of what it recommends you bring in for yourself and the baby.

bag for labor

◎ Labor aids might include: music and a tape or CD; massage oil; birth ball; massage roller (or rolling pin or tennis ball); a spray bottle for spraying water and an aromatherapy refresher; lip balm; plenty of food and drink for your labor support person or people (you don't want to have to do without them while they go out hunter-gathering) and sustaining snacks for yourself; warm socks and slippers; glucose sweets or sugar-free lollipops; aromatherapy oils.

◎ Bring something to wear such as a large T-shirt, giant-sized cotton shirt, or cotton nightie. If you want to keep some semblance of being covered up during labor, go for a front-buttoning shirt (or back-to-front hospital gown) so you can have easy skin-to-skin contact and breastfeed your baby after delivery. Whatever you labor in is likely to get stuff all over it: whoever does your washing should soak clothing with blood stains in cold water before throwing it in the washing machine. You might also need a couple of pairs of dark undies and some pads to absorb leaking amniotic fluid while you're in labor.

◎ Pack toiletries—soap, shampoo, conditioner, toothbrush, and toothpaste, moisturizer, hair elastics, hairbrush, hair dryer, shower cap—ear plugs, eye mask, and makeup if you want to clean up a bit for visitors.

◎ The support person's clothes should be comfortable, not too warm, and easy to wash. If your support person is likely to be, for instance, giving you pain relief massage in the shower, they might also want to pack a bathing suit, because hospitals do try to restrict the number of people running around in the nudey-rudey.

◎ Apparently some people who are into "creative visualization" look at a photo of their dog. Of course they're obviously insane.

a bigger bag for the hospital stay

⊚ Include a few front-opening nighties, a robe, slippers, six pairs of black cotton undies. It would be nice to have a clean nightie each morning and each night, and plenty of cotton undies—it's a leaky old time. You can wear regular day clothes in hospital, but the combination of a sore, tender, and tired body, and the number of times you'll need access to the business end makes cotton nighties a practical choice.

⊚ Bring at least two well-fitting nursing bras for supporting tight, engorged breasts, and nursing pads to soak up the leaking breast milk when it comes in.

⊚ Pack going-home clothes for you (probably maternity clothes because your tummy will still be big) and for the baby—include a hat and a warm blanket if the weather's cold. New babies love to be wrapped up firmly because it's more womblike—flannel receiving blankets are ideal for this purpose.

⊚ Bring a few super-soaker sanitary pads for the ride home.

⊚ Take a newborn-baby-care book such as *The Baby Book* by William and Martha Sears, or *What to Expect in the First Year*, by Arlene Eisenberg and cohorts (see Baby-Care Books in Week 43), and a book of names if that debate is still dragging on.

⊚ Don't forget a wrapped present for your toddler so they feel central to the action. This is the beginning of a difficult time for them, and they will be nicer to the new baby if they think it's brought them a special present.

WEEK 34

wandering Hands

what's going on

From now on your baby will hog all available space and squash up anything silly enough to get in the way, like your lungs. If you do get breathless, sitting or standing up straight will help. So will taking it easy. If you're interested in going to childbirth classes but haven't organized this yet, you'd better make that phone call now. Lay in the "layette" (baby's clothes).

Your body is starting to put the final touches to the baby: it's the finishing-school stage. From now on your bub is pretty busy practicing sucking, breathing, blinking, turning the head, grabbing things (such as its other hand or the umbilical cord), and stretching out the legs—but there's not quite enough room to actually do that. Hence the jarring kicks you may feel. The baby's skin is becoming smoother and less translucent—more like the final skin color.

Weight: about 4 1/2 pounds.

Average approximate baby length this week from head to butt

7   8   9   10   11

DiARY

It's really hard to find comfy positions. If I lean back, I get heartburn. If I lean forward, I'm not resting, I'm listing. If I lie down, I can't get anything done. If I don't lie down, the fluid retention reaches epic proportions. If I lie down, my lower legs ache. If I walk around, I aggravate an ache in my groin. At the start of the day my face is all puffy. By the end of the day my ankles are all puffy. I'm starting to feel like one of those ballpoint pens with the liquid in the side: if you turn it upside down all the liquid falls down and the girl's bikini top comes off. Now I can't even adequately describe a novelty souvenir writing implement.

Make the mistake of trying to buy a dress in a swank boutique with three mirrors in the dressing room. When I realize what I look like from behind, I have to sit down on it for a minute, in shock. And my arms look like the sort of arms that gigantic ladies get a few years after their wood-chopping days are over. Good grief.

I skitter between nausea and indigestion and faintness and wondering if that weird feeling is hunger.

This baby is a kicker. I try to imagine what else it will be like when it comes out. Still trying to get past the thoughts of labor itself, and wondering how on earth I can get all my work finished before the Blini arrives.

Matt finally cleans up his room but leaves all his water polo trophies on the mantelpiece. There is a rather tension-ridden scene with me trying to be diplomatic ("How would you feel if we put your trophies up in the living room?") and Matt looking grumpy. Perhaps it is some deep-seated male displacement thing going on. Poor Matt. He gets his own back by doing a load of new baby things in the wash (to make sure there are no manufacturing chemicals left on them) and waving a very tiny sock at me, which he knows perfectly well will reduce me to tears.

A tree in the backyard drops a big branch. A tree "surgeon" (why not "barber"?) comes and describes it jauntily as "self-lopping," so of course now we have to cut down a perfectly charming tree full of birds and expose ourselves to the scrutiny of approximately ninety berzillion apartments in the block behind because we don't

want it self-lopping onto the baby. And that will be $200, thanks.
Honestly sometimes you don't know where the next bill is
coming from.

Aunt Peg is now worried about dust in the baby's room.

"It's thoroughly dusted and vacuumed once a week," I reassure
her. Well, that's a lie.

You don't so much reassure her as send her fleeing to another
fixation.

"There'll still be dust in there," she warns ominously, as if the
dust were somehow radioactive.

Then when I say I am looking for a woollen blanket or shawl to
wrap the baby in when it's cold, she starts in about that.

"I don't understand," she says, muttering about heat stroke
and meningitis and the fall of civilization as we know it. "Nobody I
know wraps a baby in a wool blanket. They might throw one onto
the stroller, but it's not for wrapping up."

"Yes, okay," I finally say. "I'll just throw it on the stroller, then."

Oops. Just remembered we don't have a stroller. Must call
Luke and Fatimah to claim theirs.

Buy some extra-large pajamas to take to the hospital. Start to
pack hospital bag. The top of the pajamas doesn't even look like
it will fit me now, and as they were mail order I didn't realize
they were going to say "Brand New Mom" on the pocket. How
ostentatious. And I think that will be fairly obvious without anyone
having to read my pajama pocket. Especially because the guy who
designed the Brand New Mom's pajamas didn't leave enough
room for a not-yet-deflated tummy. You'd think someone in the
fashion industry would know better . . . I must have totally lost my
marbles: I could have gotten one of the seamstresses at work to
run up a giant T-shirt in 4 minutes flat.

This gum nodule thing just above my front teeth seems to be
getting worse. It bleeds profusely every time I brush my teeth and
is clearly visible as a kind of bulge between two teeth. I have
started to spit blood like a prizefighter. The only book that
mentions it is *What to Expect When You're Expecting*, which says it's
called a pyogenic granuloma, or in the usual deeply reassuring

doctor language a "pregnancy tumor," which is actually
completely harmless and will go away right after the baby's born.
Which is not what my dentist says.

My dentist says (after inquiring whether the baby's father is my
boyfriend or my husband, a question obviously essential to dental
hygiene): "It won't go away. I can just slice it off. It will bleed for
an hour or so and then be all right."

Call me crazy, but I'm going to wait and see.*

Everyone is saying how beautiful Marg's baby is. I am starting
to feel a bit paranoid that our baby will be as ugly as a dog and
there will just be polite silences on the subject.

I have been thinking about the birth plan and I've decided
that I don't want the baby to come out the vagina, and I don't
want a cesarean. I may have to do some more research. Perhaps it
can come out of an elbow.

The waistbands of my pants have started rolling down all of
their own accord.

I'm too busy to have a child.

Walk to work and get completely exhausted. Business lunch
follows. Try to be sparkling and feel like I'm mentally swimming
in pudding.

Miss my appointment with Dr. Herb as he is out delivering a
baby somewhere, and I can't face the waiting room locked up with
trillions of tired women so I don't show up.

I am SO huge out the front that close friends can't help just
patting and rubbing my tummy—like I'm a Buddha—for luck.
I don't mind. People have started to ask "How long to go?," and
"Are you excited?" (some kind of code word for "utterly terrified,"
perhaps).

The last childbirth class: by this stage all the people in the class
who were going to loosen up have loosened up. Only two couples
haven't lost their quiet, stunned approach to everything. One
woman keeps looking at her partner as if he's a ghastly apparition
and she's suddenly realized she's tied to him for the rest of her life.

The picture I'll take with me is of women bulging in the
middle, with their hands crossed over their bulge and their male

* The book was right.

partner leaning toward them. The woman who wanted her birth on the Internet, and her husband, the filthy show-offs, arrive halfway through the class, with their baby! It came 2 weeks early, on the weekend, and they're still high. Melissa confides that she doesn't let parents come if they've hit the baby-blues stage. You don't want a brand-new mother sobbing and falling about a class, I suppose.

Melissa shows us two videos of couples with new babies. The men all work away from home and the women at home. The couples talk about lack of privacy and personal space, their relationship as a couple, tiredness, guilt, coping with a distressed and needy baby (the gist seems to be that "this too shall pass"). And there's footage of a woman with twins: she looks a bit like someone has hit her on the back of the head with a plastic baseball bat. You would, wouldn't you?

Melissa talks about having a baby who cries a lot. New ones sleep 16 hours a day, but after a few weeks or months they can cry for a few hours a day no matter how well fed and clean and cuddled they are. This is often in the early evening and is known as the "witching hour." Many women say there's a crying "peak" at about 6 weeks old.

We gallop through some different things to settle the baby; how not to expect much from your sex life until at least after the 6-week checkup (one man mishears and shouts "Six years?!"); contraception (twelve condoms at once, thank you); services available if you get into trouble with feeding, sleeping, or crying; and baby safety.

Revelation: one woman in the class asks, "Shouldn't you have the baby checked out by a pediatrician before it goes home?" Melissa says yes, most parents do. I haven't even thought of this. I guess the obstetrician is a mother specialist, not a baby specialist.

info

labor

You might or might not notice the early signs of labor. If you do, rest and eat—labor could start any time and you need to conserve your energy, though the Real Thing may still be up to a few days or even weeks away.

When your contractions start, they may be prelabor, sometimes called false contractions. These are quite bearable—more uncomfortable than painful—and irregular, and they go away if you move around, lie down, or have a bath. It's often difficult to tell the difference between prelabor and the latent phase of the first stage of labor (during which the cervix dilates 3–4 centimeters), so don't hesitate to telephone your midwife, the hospital or birth center, or your obstetrician to describe what's happening and to find out whether to stay at home or go straight to the hospital or center.

Call your hospital or obstetrician immediately if:

☉ your water breaks.

☉ you have bright red bleeding, which may indicate a problem with the placenta.

☉ you feel or see the umbilical cord in your vagina, which is called cord prolapse. This is an emergency. Call 911, open the door, then kneel down with your bottom in the air and head and shoulders down to take pressure off the cord until the ambulance arrives. (If you can, get someone else to make the call and open the door.)

DESTINATION UNKNOWN

When contractions start in earnest, they will usually:

⊚ be regular.

⊚ get stronger.

⊚ last longer.

⊚ come closer together.

⊚ be increasingly tough to cope with.

Time their length and frequency and give this information to your obstetrician or midwife, or the hospital or birth center.

The average labor *for a first-timer* goes something like this:

⊚ first stage—the cervix dilates to 8–9 centimeters (average 8 hours).

⊚ first stage transition (second part of the first stage)—the cervix dilates to about 10 centimeters (can be 3–5 hours).

⊚ second stage—buildup to pushing, then the baby is born (average 2 hours).

⊚ third stage—the placenta and any other bits no longer needed are expelled (about 20 minutes after the birth if pitocin is given, up to an hour if delivered naturally).

Gosh, that sounds neat. In reality your experience might be radically different.

When you arrive at the hospital or birth center, or when the midwife or obstetrician arrives for your home birth, you'll have a medical examination, which will probably involve:

⊚ checking your blood pressure.

⊚ checking a urine sample.

⊚ checking your temperature and pulse.

⊚ a feel up your vagina to see how dilated your cervix is.

⑥ electronic monitoring of the baby's heartbeat, usually done by placing a belt around your tummy, which is attached by wires to a machine that prints out when your uterus contracts and also records the baby's heartbeat. The monitor is often removed after a set time (for example, 20 minutes) if there seems to be no problem.

Make sure the midwife or nurse makes a note of your relevant health details or special needs.

Ideally things will now proceed according to your birth plan. But any unpredictable turns will have to be dealt with as they arise.

first stage

For some people the latent phase of first-stage labor—the first 3–4 centimeters dilation—is barely perceptible; others experience intense backache and painful contractions. For some it happens quietly over a long time; for others it may all happen in just a couple of hours of full-on labor. Contractions may last 30–35 seconds and can be regular or irregular—anywhere from 5 to 20 minutes apart. You'll probably be at home and may even be able to sleep through some of this phase. Rest as much as possible and have some of the light snacks you have ready in the freezer. It can help to have warm baths, if your waters haven't broken, and you should keep timing your contractions.

All the following advice may fly out of your head, so get your birth support person to read it well before you might need it so that they can remind you.

By the time you're well into the first stage, you'll probably be in the hospital and looking to your coping strategies: massage, relaxation techniques, breathing techniques. Not to mention drugs. Remember to pee frequently: the area is feeling such intense sensations from labor that you mightn't notice you need to pee. Stay as mobile and upright as possible. Try out different laboring positions for greatest comfort. Stay hydrated, taking ice chips, juice popsicles, or sips of water.

Try to completely rest and relax between contractions, and not expend energy anticipating the next one. Use positive visualization and psyching techniques, such as concentrating on a mental picture of a flower opening; focus on the positive goal of seeing your baby; chant "This will end," or whatever. Clenching everything up can hinder the progress of labor, so with your partner or labor support person's help use whatever it takes to go with the flow. If you can't stand the pain, or if this phase has gone on for a long time and you've had it, feel free to yell "DRUGS!" around about now.

first stage transition

This is generally considered to be the most challenging time of labor. Contractions are strong and getting stronger, lasting longer—60–90 seconds—and coming at shorter intervals. Sometimes there's no time to rest between them, and you're probably exhausted. You may feel hot or shivering and cold, or alternate between temperature extremes. You may be nauseated or vomiting and feeling overwhelmed or unable to cope. You may feel totally pissed off.

At the end of this phase your cervix will be fully dilated, and you'll be ready to start pushing. If you've hung in there without drugs, your support person can remind you that you are nearly there, that you'll have your baby very soon, and you can hit your support person. If you have the urge to push during this phase, before the cervix is fully dilated, you may be advised to blow or pant instead.

second stage—pushing and delivery

About a third of laboring women have a resting, or latent, phase at this point before their body starts urging them to push the baby out—the active phase of the second stage. The goal during this phase is to listen to your body when it comes to pushing. Contractions will still be 60–90 seconds long but may be farther apart (2–5 minutes), so you can rest between them. No need to pop the capillaries in your eyeballs or hold your breath beyond the point of comfort or turn purple. Using lots of shorter moments of bearing down with each contraction is less stressful to the baby and makes it easier for the pelvic floor to relax, than one big, breath-holding push, like the ones you see in the movies.

This more relaxed approach may make the second stage a bit longer but it is probably less stressful for you as well as the baby. During this phase you might be making some deep guttural grunts and moans, which many other pregnancy books seem to think will embarrass you. You'll be far too busy to be embarrassed. You might also push out a poop during this phase. No big deal.

All being well, babies are not oxygen-deprived during this phase; they're still getting oxygen from the placenta.

Actual, honest-to-goodness birth   There's more panting as the baby's head crowns and pushes against the perineum. You'll be asked to try not to push but instead to relax the pelvic floor, aiming to slow down the last bit to avoid tearing or the need for an episiotomy. You may be offered a bird's-eye view of the proceedings with the help of a mirror: this is a fascinating prospect for some, and horrifying for others. You choose.

Moms often describe the sensation of the baby's head emerging as stinging, burning, or intense pressure. After the head emerges, the baby rotates so that its shoulders line up with the widest part of your pelvis and the little body slithers out. Hello there! Finally meeting and holding your baby is an indescribably awe-inspiring, emotional, and happy time. (Or not, of which more later.)

third stage: the placenta and membranes expelled

You may be so engrossed in your new baby, you don't notice the third stage. The uterus continues to contract, causing the placenta to come away from the wall, taking with it what's left of the amniotic sac as it detaches; further contractions will push the placenta into the vagina, from where it can be pulled out, or pushed out with another contraction. The contraction of the muscles of your truly amazing uterus also seals off the blood vessels at the site of detachment. The placenta comes out more quickly if an injection of oxytocin is given to speed up contractions.

The placenta is inspected to make sure it has been delivered whole. You'll be checked to make sure you don't have postpartum hemorrhage (postpartum means after delivery). It's diagnosed when the blood loss is 500 milliliters or more; the usual loss is less than 400 milliliters. It happens to about 5 percent of mothers.

The fourth stage, hardly ever mentioned in the textbooks, is stabilization and getting acquainted with your baby, enjoying skin-to-skin contact, keeping your baby warm, the baby having a red-hot go and first drink at your nipples, the standard reflex and observation tests on the baby done by a doctor or midwife, clamping of the umbilical cord, and any sewing up of the perineum.

YOU MAY NEED BIGGER SHOES

WEEK 35

what's going on

That baby is taking up stomach space— smaller meals more often are easier to digest. You're probably finding it hard to get your shoes on and off. Wear slip-on shoes unless you need the ankle support of lace-ups. You've probably gone up a shoe size as well, especially in width, maybe permanently. Try to walk a bit every day until the baby arrives. To reduce the swelling in your feet and ankles, stand on your head a lot. Or at the very least sit down or, preferably, lie down and put your feet above the level of your heart as much as possible. (This can be especially effective in getting yourself extra room on public transport, particularly if you shout obscenities as well.)

Toenails are in. The fingernails may be poking over the end of the fingers. Weight: about 5 pounds.

Average approximate baby length this week from head to butt

Diary

Help, it's going too fast. I'm not ready but I'm sick of being pregnant. Bunty, who does the accounts at work, says she lost 30 pounds at the birth, including the weight of the baby, and I must say THAT'S an attractive proposition. I'm wondering how long my legs will carry me. I weigh myself at a pharmacy and it says I've put on 14 pounds in five days. God, I hope those scales are faulty. I'm terrified of getting on the scales at Dr. Herb's.

Before I leave the pharmacy the assistant thrusts into my hands the special drug store's sample bag to encourage me to come back and buy baby stuff there. You get your nursing pads (colostrum-and-milk-soaker-upperers), five diaper liners (whatever *they* are), twelve thick baby wipes, a disposable diaper, a sample of cocoa-butter moisturizer, a pamphlet on same, a booklet about safety, and a copy of *Practical Parenting* magazine with the cover line "I gave birth in a gas station!," which, frankly I don't think has enough exclamation marks, and what's practical about giving birth in a gas station I'd like to know.

I take an inventory of stretch marks. Several red-purple stripes on the underside of each breast, and on each hip a bunch of marks that looks as if a hand held me too hard on each fleshy part. Nothing on the tummy itself, which has stretched more than anything. What gives? Me.

Yet another visit to Dr. Herb for the fluid-retention check.

He measures the height of the baby, gives it a feel and says, "Oh God."

First "My, it's a whopper" and now "Oh God." If this goes on he'll be singing "Oh What a Beauty! Never Seen One as Big as That Befooooore!" on my next visit. For some reason I feel resigned rather than horrified. I suspect his tactic is to soften me up and get me used to the idea of a boombah bambino.

I show him the birth plan and he reacts to each point.

Will you induce at the due date? (No. I'll let you go ten days over.)

Ideally I would like to avoid either a vaginal birth or a cesarean. However, there do not seem to be many other options. (Ha ha. By hook or by crook the baby will come out.)

The labor will be attended by my doula, Miss Beck, who will probably prescribe herbs and supplements after the birth. (Fine.)

I would like to be kept informed of what's happening. (Yep.)

I would like to avoid monitoring that might "tether" me to the bed, and an epidural, if possible. Matt is particularly concerned about the possible side effects of an epidural, but understands it might not be avoidable. Anyway it's my decision. (It certainly is.)

I would like to avoid an episiotomy, but would rather be cut than tear if necessary. (Although sometimes an episiotomy is unavoidable, we will try to avoid it. Actually it's better to tear naturally unless it looks like you're going to tear down to the bowel or up to the clitoris, or shatter the whole area, which is hard to repair.) (Me: That's enough. Fine. That's quite enough chat about torn clitorises for one day.)

I don't want gas, would rather take Demerol. (You should try the gas, and see if it works.) (Me: No way—haven't you seen that movie *Blue Velvet*, where Dennis Hopper has this mask on and . . .) (No.)

My Major Fears, in order, are:

1. possible neurological damage from epidural. (About the same chance as getting hit by a jumbo jet, unless you already have a history of trouble, such as multiple sclerosis.)

2. episiotomy. (You and I will just keep in contact throughout the delivery.)

But generally we agree: whatever it takes to get a healthy baby out with the least amount of damage possible all round.

While Herb is checking my blood pressure, I remark that it doesn't seem to be within the laws of physics, but I appear to have put on another 8 pounds. At least Dr. Herb's scales say I'm 6 pounds lighter than the pharmacist's did. I think I'm going to explode. This means I have put on 40 pounds!!! I'm not eating crap—in fact I'm not eating a lot at all. It's spooky.

Dr. Herb says don't worry, I'll probably put on another 10 pounds before I give birth. I am absolutely flabbergasted.

"It's not humanly possible," I say.

"Don't forget," he says, "you can lose 24 pounds just at the birth, and all the fluid over the next couple of weeks. Of course you can actually puff up after the birth as well. You'll lose it. It's easier to lose the weight that's not junk food."

I don't tell him I have at least three Haagen Dazs a week.

Marg has given me a book called *The New Age Baby Name Book* by Susan Browder. Could its names be worse than some of the suggestions from friends so far, including Hezekiah, Ringo, or Bluey if it's a boy. And if it's a girl, geographical names such as India, Georgia, and, what's next, Grand Canyon? How about fabric names such as Chiffon, Polly Esther, and Tencel?

I guess I have to remember that I come from a family that has definite trouble with names. My grandmother named her three daughters after whatever household item she was holding at the time she went into labor: Peg, Bobbin, and Rose. (Thank God she was gardening for the last one and not cleaning the bathroom or Mom would have been called Toilet Brush.)

There's some very good advice in the book, which you would already know unless you were completely brain dead, such as: if you have twin boys don't call them Pete and Repeat because the joke will wear off. It mentions a man in San Francisco who became a circus clown (naturally) whose real name was Oofty Goofty Bowman. Matt and I are thrilled and immediately rename the Blini Oofty Goofty.

According to *The New Age Baby Name Book*, in some cultures they name kids for what time of the day or night they arrive. Luckily this has not caught on here, where not many children are called Sparrow's Fart or Half Past Three. And you can use the

Ghanaian language to call the child after the day of the week it was born on. Young Wednesday from *The Addams Family* would have been called Ekua.

You can also use any unfamiliar language to name your baby after a certain characteristic. What is the Burkina Fasoese for "reluctant to mow the lawn," I wonder.

The book goes so far as to advise using the name Caimile from the Umbundu people of Africa, which is a sort of code for the proverb "A tree bears fruit, the fruit falls to the ground, a family has children, and they all die." How jaunty. And it suggests stealing some Native American names even if you're not, such as Helkimu, meaning "hitting bushes with seed beater." I think it would be better to wait and see whether the child grew up to be interested in whacking bushes before putting that kind of pressure on it.

I don't think Yuttciso is going to catch on. It means "lice thick on a chicken hawk." The book says American names that have fallen out of favor include Minnehaha, Amorous, Ham, Lettuce, and Bugless.

The book has also translated some names from their original Celtic meanings. Calvin Klein, for instance, means "young, small, bald man." And Mary Tyler Moore means "bitter, dark-skinned roofer."

But the handiest idea of them all is just to combine the names of the parents. For example, if your names are Mel and Trisha, you can call the kid Militia. Or, say, if your names are Louise and Arnie, you can call it Loonie. It's easy. Paul and May Ling?—Appalling. Bathsheba and Matthew?—Bath matt. And in our case, Madmatt. Sounds like some kind of deranged criminal.

I have learned that we should only ever try out our suggested names on a few friends. There'll always be someone who doesn't like the name you choose because there was a girl at their kindergarten called that who used to put paste in their hair. Or it was the name of the first man who dumped them. Best to just hit them with a fait accompli after the kid's born, and they'll have to put on a brave face and get used to it.

more info on baby names

The New Age Baby Name Book by Susan Browder,
Warner Books, New York, 1987.

An unintentionally hilarious, list of absolutely insanely
stupid names you could give your child, as well as some
definite possibilities. Good for seeing names from
different cultures. It ranges from Agnes to Zaim, meaning
"brigadier-general" in Arabic.

info

cesarean delivery

A cesarean section operation is a surgical procedure to take the baby out of
the uterus through your abdomen. It's
usually called just "a cesarean" or "a c-
section." A standard cesarean is
considered to be a very safe
procedure when performed
by a specialist in a good
hospital. But it is not a walk in
the park. A cesarean is major
surgery. (The way some people blithely
refer to it, you'd think the baby just came
out of a handy zipper.)

how common is it?

Depending on several factors, your chance
of having a cesarean might be a lot
greater than you think. About 22
percent of American babies are delivered this way. Read up on it
because it might happen to you, even if you've had a "perfect"
pregnancy.

what happens?

During a standard cesarean, you may have the top half of your pubic hair trimmed or shaved, and then you'll be put on a hospital gurney and wheeled off to the operating room. In this very brightly lit room all the medical staff will wear sterile caps, face masks, and protective smocks, and so will your support person. An intravenous (IV) drip will be put into your arm, then you'll be given an epidural injection (or spinal-block injection) by the anesthesiologist (explained in Pain Relief Options in Week 32) to numb the lower half of your body. As well, a catheter tube will be put into your urethra for the urine to flow into a bag. A screen will be put up between your upper body and your tummy. If there is the need for general anesthesia, your support person may not be allowed in the operating room.

A nurse will swab the lower part of your tummy with antiseptic. Your obstetrician will make an incision just above your pubic hairline, usually horizontal and about 10 centimeters long. Then the obstetrician will cut through layers of fat and muscle to the uterus wall, cut open the uterus, and pull the baby out. You may have some sensation of pulling or pressure but should feel no pain.

It all happens very quickly: the baby is generally born about 10 minutes after the first incision. The baby will be shown to you after being assessed by the pediatric team in the operating room. The baby might also have mucous sucked from its tiny airways. If the baby doesn't need to be taken away for special care, have a long cuddle. Often the baby will then go to the nursery for observation. You may ask to keep the baby with you. Many hospitals take babies away to suit their policy, not you.

You might be too preoccupied to notice what happens next, but usually the placenta and membranes, are removed, then you are stitched up. This can take quite a while because it's not just one row of stitches, it's many different layers to be sewn, including layers of skin, fat, muscle, and the inner and outer walls of the uterus.

why would you need one?

A cesarean can be elective: you "elect" to have one on the advice of your obstetrician and make a hospital appointment. Or it can be emergency surgery performed unexpectedly and suddenly when a problem develops during labor. In the case of an elective cesarean, you have to weigh the pros and cons of setting a date rather than waiting for the spontaneous onset of labor. These can be discussed with your obstetrician and midwife.

If you want to avoid having a cesarean, talk to your obstetrician, but remember that there's never a guarantee you won't have one.

The basic criterion for a cesarean is whether it will be less of a risk to the mother and baby than a vaginal birth. In some cases the decision is very clear-cut; in others it's more open to interpretation. Some reasons why you might end up needing a cesarean are:

⑥ you have a medical condition such as preeclampsia or eclampsia (see info in Week 31).

⑥ active genital herpes (the baby may catch the herpes from sores as it comes through the vagina).

⑥ the baby is sick or isn't growing properly.

⑥ the baby is in an awkward position—perhaps sideways, which is known as the "transverse lie," or with its butt not head down, which is called the "breech position" (some obstetricians will agree to try first to deliver a breech baby in the normal way).

⑥ the baby's head seems to be too big to fit through its mom's pelvis; this is technically called cephalopelvic disproportion (CPD).

⑥ placenta previa (the placenta is positioned over the cervix).

⑥ placental abruption (the placenta comes away too early).

⑥ an overdue baby in a deteriorating uterine environment.

⑥ the umbilical cord is "prolapsed"—coming down into the vagina, possibly cutting off the baby's circulation if the baby's head is against the cervix.

⑥ the baby's lowered or erratic heartbeat during labor indicates it is distressed or in danger.

⑥ failure to progress during labor.

recovery from the surgery

Probably the first thing you'll notice when you're in the recovery room or back in your own hospital room is that you're still hooked up to the IV drip and peeing into a bag through a tube, which will continue for up to a day. Once you are settled in the recovery room, ask to have the baby for a breastfeeding session. Often a long-lasting morphine medication has been placed in the epidural or spinal block helping to reduce your pain for the first 24 hours. Otherwise, you may get injections of pain medications through your IV. There is no reason for you to have severe or moderate pain. Talk to your nurse or doctor if you need more pain medication.

Over several days your pain is likely to be reduced. Don't skimp on relief, and ask the nurses or midwives for it if they miss your due time or you are in pain. It's important not to be in pain whenever possible.

See or call your naturopath about any vitamins and minerals that may help recovery. Make sure they're approved for lactation and by your doctor.

Get up and move as soon as humanly possible. Immediately after you can feel your legs again, start flexing and rotating your feet, and doing leg bends in bed. Get out of bed and go for a walk as soon as you're allowed to. It won't be a brisk hike, mind you. It'll be more of a small shuffle around the bed. Soon you'll be going down the corridor and back. Make sure someone goes with you because you'll be a bit woozy.

Early mobility will help you to avoid complications such as pain from gas, difficulty peeing, and blood clots in the legs. And it's amazing how quickly you start to feel better once you are mobile. But DON'T OVERDO IT. Do only half as much as you feel you can, even if you're sure you can walk around the whole block on day 4. Discipline yourself to increase the exercise a *little* bit each day, otherwise you'll get overtired and set back your recovery.

Laughing, coughing, and sneezing in bed are less painful if you bend your knees and support your scar with a pillow. If you're standing up, bend over and put your hands over the scar. Avoid constipation, as it will be painful. If it gets to dire proportions (4 to 5 days without a poop) your doctor can prescribe an anal suppository.

Your tummy will look as if it's in the earlier stages of pregnancy for a while. It will be sore, but on the plus side there will be no stitches in your vagina.

Your hospital stay will be longer than for a vaginal delivery—3–5 days, depending on hospital policy and how you feel. Don't be swayed by friends or staff—if you want to go earlier or stay longer, discuss it with your obstetrician and do the best thing for you. You should probably check with your insurance company to see whether a longer stay will be covered. After you go home, any sign of infection such as oozing, fever, or increasing pain should, of course, be reported to your obstetrician.

Full recovery is generally longer term than for vaginal delivery—it's about 6 weeks until everything is healed up and several more weeks before you're up to full pre-pregnancy exercise capabilities. And, of course, it is harder to look after a baby and recover from major abdominal surgery at the same time. You will be very tired, and your body will be in shock for longer. Remember that recovering from a cesarean is comparable to convalescing after a serious car accident: go easy on yourself.

The double burden of looking after a baby and recovering from surgery can lead to feelings of depression and some women believe they are "failures" because they have not had a natural birth. Having a c-section, though, doesn't necessarily mean you'll have negative feelings about the birth—not least because it may have saved your life or the baby's.

You're usually told not to drive until your 6-week checkup (mainly because it hurts to brake so you may brake more slowly than usual), although some doctors believe it is safe after about 3 weeks. You're also usually told not to lift anything heavier than your baby, before the 6-week checkup. The rules for taking things easy still apply: only do half of the exercise you think you can do, and keep it gentle.

more info on cesareans

 Childbirth Choices by Adriene Bennett, Wendi Etherington, and Daphne Hewson, and **Your Baby and the Birth Experience** by Dr. Gregory Fox (full details and reviews in Week 32).

Both these books cover cesarean deliveries in detail.

what's going on

You're tired. You've probably got sore feet, fluid retention causing swollen everything, and tingling fingers, and you could be breathless or dizzy. If you're really lucky you might even faint. You may get stabbing pelvic pains or aches—like a stitch—which are probably the pelvic ligaments loosening up. The baby's head may be down low in the pelvis and can bounce up and down on your cervix giving you "shocks," particularly if you sit down too quickly. This doesn't necessarily mean that the baby is "engaged" (in position and ready to come out headfirst). You should be feeling movements every day, even if it's only a little leg wave.

Those new lungs are still not completely finished. The baby has put on lots of fat. If it hasn't turned upside down already, it may be about to. (If it's still the wrong way up by the time labor starts, you may have a breech birth—meaning bottom first.) Weight: about 5¹/₂ pounds.

EK 36

lungs (2)

stomach

pancreas

uterus

Pacific
Ocean

DiaGRaM of KeY ORGaNS
iN LaTe PReGNaNCY

Average approximate baby length this week from head to butt

DiARY

Wish I had given up work. The boss wants me to fly to another city for a business meeting. Fat chance. Ha. That would be a hollow laugh except that I feel anything but hollow. Instead of waddling, I now lurch from side to side like a drunken Yeti.

On the way up to my doctor's appointment (I have to go every week in the last month), a woman in the elevator tells me she had a 1-hour labor and not to worry, it doesn't even hurt. I think she might have been at the Demerol cabinet. Dr. Herb says I'm still "carrying high".

"I'd bet that you won't go early," he says.

He reminds me I'll probably put on another 10 pounds.

The lumps that come and go in my armpit have nothing to do with deodorant, he says. They're actually breast tissue getting overexcited about soon having to produce milk and are called "breast tails." Which sounds like a stripper's specialty to me.

Aunt Peg is making cushions (don't ask me why). Uncle Stan is calling up to see how I'm going. Just had a horrible vision of Aurelia and Aunt Peg meeting over the head of the new baby in the hospital. Must warn Uncle Stan to keep Aurelia away until we come home. Keeping Aunt Peg away would be possible only with a very cunning plan and some heavy security at the perimeter.

Finally surrendering to the inevitable and taking on the role of Muhammad trying to escape the mountain, Matt is sleeping on the couch.

My old pal Simon Weaselpantz has scoured the county fairs and sent the little Blini a knitted bear and a knitted bunny rabbit. Thank heavens some people are keeping up the old skills. Women used to know how to do "fancy work," showing-off sewing, crocheting, knitting, tatting, and heaven knows what else. Now they're lucky if they know how to order a caffe latte for themselves. Can't say I would like to go back to the old days, but nice to know somebody is keeping up appearances.

Jill is organizing a baby shower for me and helping me compile a database for the birth announcements. We've got two versions ready to go, one that says Eddy and one that says Pearl. I think that's all the options covered. I've been thinking about the pros and cons of having a boy or a girl. Boy: won't be so bombarded with "you're ugly" messages from advertising and film and TV. Girl: will probably find it easier to talk about emotions and be slightly less likely to play noisy war games on the roof.

Although, truth be told, it's impossible to really imagine what it will be like when this baby is OUT. The baby-being-IN thing and the getting-the-baby-out thing just take up so much brain space.

The worst thing about being this pregnant, except for being uncomfortable and sort of nervous (could go any time from now), is that if you have someone to cuddle it's an exercise in geometry. It's impossible to get really close with a third person stuck way out there in the middle.

info

late babies

why are babies late?

Your baby is not likely to arrive at precisely midnight on the 266th day of pregnancy. So if it isn't early, it's going to be late (der). We don't know exactly what makes a woman's body go into labor, but it's now believed that the baby, when ready to be born, somehow releases hormones or prostaglandins or a greeting card or something that doctors don't know about yet. This unknown signal triggers the softening of the cervix, ready for it to dilate and let the baby through, and contractions of the uterus.

About 10 percent of pregnancies go over 40 weeks. Often these are first-time mothers. "They" now think that this is because the due date is often miscalculated. This would mean that true overdue pregnancies going over 42 weeks are more like 2 percent. If you go beyond 42 weeks, your doctor is likely to induce the birth.

how long can you go?

You can go up to 43 weeks with careful monitoring, although most obstetricians and midwives don't like to leave it that long. Beyond 42 weeks of pregnancy, babies are at increased risk of fetal distress during labor, inhaling their first poop, and as the placenta starts packing up, the baby could even die.

Some of the most common methods of checking that an overdue baby is okay are:

⑥ you keep a "kick chart" to monitor how much the baby is moving.

⑥ electronic monitoring of the baby's heart rate to make sure it is not distressed.

⑥ an ultrasound to help estimate the amount of amniotic fluid.

induction methods

Prostaglandins Prostaglandins (which are like hormones) are found naturally in the uterus; some prostaglandins stimulate contractions at the beginning of labor. A synthetic prostaglandin gel or suppository placed in the vagina can ripen the cervix and occasionally trigger labor. It usually takes a number of doses, sometimes spaced over more than a day, before the cervix is ripened enough to start IV pitocin, which will start the labor contractions.

Artificial rupture of the membranes (amniotomy) A plastic hook called an amniohook (sort of like a slim crochet hook) is used to break the membranes of the amniotic sac. Often it is enough just to brush the hook against the membranes, but sometimes it will have to be inserted to make a small hole. It usually doesn't hurt at all. Once the membranes have been broken, labor usually follows quickly as the baby's head is no longer cushioned by amniotic fluid and so descends, putting pressure on the ripe cervix and encouraging it to widen. Breaking the membranes also triggers the release of prostaglandins, which help to speed up the labor process.

Artificial rupture of the membranes is a very effective method of induction on its own if the cervix is ripe. Amniotomy is often used during an otherwise normal labor to speed things up, and also if an electrode needs to be attached to your baby's scalp to monitor its heartbeat.

Pitocin A synthetic form of oxytocin (the hormone that causes the uterus to contract) is given through an IV drip to increase the strength and regularity of contractions. Contractions brought on by pictocin are usually stronger, longer, and more painful than normal, so pain relief drugs are often used during labor.

Other methods:

⊚ acupuncture or acupressure—often a course of a few treatments over a few days—which must be performed by a trained specialist.

⊚ some homoeopathic remedies can be used to help ripen the cervix—again these must be prescribed by a naturopath experienced in pregnancy care.

⊚ nipple massage—gently massage one nipple at a time (massaging both nipples at once has been shown to cause fetal distress), either by hand or with a warm, moist cloth, alternating nipples every 15 minutes for three periods of up to an hour each day, which can stimulate uterine contractions and ripen the cervix.

⊚ semen is rich in prostaglandins, which ripen the cervix—the easiest way to "administer" it is by having sex with, well, frankly, a man.

⊚ orgasm results in several strong uterine contractions; it is thought that these, combined with sexual arousal, can stimulate prostaglandin production.

◎ keeping moving—keeping upright and moving will allow a little extra pressure to be exerted on your cervix by your baby's head, which may stimulate ripening, but remember not to overdo it.

◎ visualization—some people believe that the power of suggestion can affect the body. If you're good at this sort of thing, try to relax and visualize the birth (leaving out any bits that make you anxious). Some women have found that watching films of babies being born triggers labor (remember all those stories about *Three Men and a Baby*?)

characteristic features of late babies
Late babies often look a bit different from those born on time.

◎ They are sometimes described as looking "overcooked" because during their extra time in the uterus they lose fat from all over their body, and their skin becomes red and wrinkly and may "crack" as the waxy coating of vernix disappears.

◎ They tend to have longer fingernails and more hair.

◎ Although often skinnier, they keep growing in the uterus so they are larger all over than babies born earlier.

◎ A longer time spent in the uterus may result in a greenish staining of the skin and umbilical cord by meconium: in very post-term babies these stains will be yellow.

your record

What labor issues do you feel really strongly about?

How do you feel about medical intervention?
What if it becomes necessary?

What have you included in your birth plan?

what's going on

Your bosoms may have developed a mind of their own and be leaking for no apparent reason or when a baby cries. (Any old baby will do.) The stuff is the colostrum, which will give your newborn baby protein and antibodies in the few days before your milk "comes in." The baby can't tumble around so much because it's run out of room, but the kicking and whacking can have a real force when they do happen. From here on in, try to be strict about getting as much rest and sleep as you can. Labor and recovery are much easier if you are well rested.

WEEK

The baby isn't doing much except putting on more weight. The tiny lungs are getting ready to work on their own. The baby has a firm hand grip and is swallowing about 24 ounces of amniotic fluid a day. Weight: about 6 pounds.

Diary — Dr. Herb says, "Don't have the baby on Saturday." He is going for his motorcycle license. He says his helmet is very black and racy. I say if I do go into labor he'll have to come, but he can wear his helmet.

"It's part of my midlife crisis," he says cheerily.

It is a measure of the serenity of Dr. Herb that this statement doesn't make me nervous in the slightest.

"Does your wife just laugh at you?" I ask.

"Yes, she does, actually."

I am not astonished.

Dr. Herb is still convinced that the Blini won't come early, but on the due date or later.

"Is it engaged?" he asks.

How would I know? All I can report is that it appears to be wearing Doc Martens and doing Irish dancing on my cervix.

I have been overcome by an ineluctable torpor. In other words I lie on the couch and watch *The Bold and the Beautiful,* and it is pointless to try doing otherwise. My priorities are all changing ("Forget all of you at work! And the horse you rode in on!"), I am consumed by stupidity hormones, and I can't seem to call people back.

I hear from Aunt Zelda, the adventuress, now settled in Botswana, who sends me a tiny card with twelve teensy buttons sewn onto it, each half the size of a little fingernail. "A decent aunt would have made these buttons into a three-piece Lafayette or something. I've had them for 20 years," she writes. I am somehow pleased she doesn't know the difference between layette and Lafayette: neither do I.

I hit the wall and give up work. I had planned to work until the first contractions, but something has happened to my brain. I was working too hard for contemplation, and my mind was demanding space. So of course what always happens when you stop working? I get a cold.

I buy some candy to put in the labor bag for energy and eat it all by 3 o'clock. I have written down the phone numbers of the hospital and Matt's work and Dr. Herb, but if I don't pin them to the inside of my underpants I'll probably lose them all.

Beck asks am I bonding with the baby? "As much as I can with someone I haven't met yet," I think. Other moms have warned me there might be an ambivalent fog descending after the birth. We'll see.

Nausea. Walks not. Horizontal. No verbs in sentences.

info

your newborn baby

Newborn babies can look pretty weird. Yours might have the following:

⑥ blood and creamy vernix all over it (premature babies have more, late babies may have hardly any).

⑥ puffy, bruised, or squinty-looking eyes.

⑥ a puffy face.

⑥ a head that looks elongated or cone-shaped because it's been squeezed through the pelvis and vagina—this will normalize, often within hours, although it can take up to a couple of weeks (the bones have spaces between them called fontanelles so that they can squish up during childbirth; these harden within several months and become one thick skull).

⑥ an unfocused, sometimes cross-eyed gaze; at this early stage a newborn can only focus on something very close, like a nipple in front of its face.

⑥ a swollen lump on the head, caused by the vacuum.

⑥ temporary indentations on the face or head or pointy-headed look from forceps.

☺ lanugo on the body—the downy hair is often across the shoulders, on the back, and on the face around the hairline (with more if the baby is premature)—which usually rubs off within a few weeks.

☺ small white spots, like pimples, on the face, which are called milia and are caused by temporary blockages of the sebaceous glands.

☺ red blotches (often called "stork bites" because they look as if a stork has held the baby in its bill) (yeah, right) on the back of the neck at the base of the skull, the forehead, and/or the eyelids, which are caused by little veins close to the skin—they will disappear after a year or so and only reappear with heat and stress, such as tantrums, during childhood.

☺ "Mongolian spots"—bluish gray patches on the back, the buttocks and sometimes the arms and thighs, which are more common in Asian and darker-skinned babies; the spots will fade away.

☺ other birthmarks (see a pediatrician if you're concerned about a birthmark).

☺ jaundice—more than half of all newborn babies become jaundiced (yellow) about 3 to 4 days after birth, but the baby's liver soon deals with this pigment, caused by the breaking down of unneeded red cells, and only a very small percentage of babies need treatment with extra fluids, sun, or ultraviolet lights to improve.

☺ big, swollen baby genitals and breasts, a discharge from the nipples, or even some blood from the baby vagina, due to a temporary oversupply of estrogen.

☺ testicles that may not yet have descended.

☺ a bruised bottom and very swollen genitals, if it's a breech-birth baby born vaginally.

routine medical stuff

The APGAR test will be performed to assess the baby's health. Named after its originator, Dr. Virginia Apgar (oh my God, something's named after a woman), it's also an acronym for the things that are checked:

◎ **a**ppearance (color).

◎ **p**ulse (heartbeat).

◎ **g**rimace (reflex).

◎ **a**ctivity (muscle tone).

◎ **r**espiration (breathing).

In each category 0, 1, or 2 points are given, and a score of 7 or more is considered to be good. The test is conducted 1 minute after birth and again 5 minutes after birth. A very low score will mean emergency medical care is needed.

It is common to suggest that all babies be given a vitamin K injection very soon after the birth as a preventative measure against hemorrhagic disease of the newborn (HDN). (If you're having a home birth, check whether the midwife will give it.) An antibiotic ointment is also often placed in the baby's eyes to prevent infection.

A full weighing, measurement of length, and medical check will include the test for congenital dislocation of the hip (CDH), which can be corrected during the first 3 months using braces or a harness to stabilize the legs while the hip joint develops.

The Guthrie or PKU test, routinely done 2 or 3 days after birth, involves a blood sample being taken from the baby's heel and is a screening test for the disorders of phenylketonuria, hypothyroidism, cystic fibrosis, and galactosemia, all of which are best caught early for treatment.

things you might not know

◎ Some newborn babies don't have tears when they cry until they are 1–3 months old.

◎ The eye color a baby's born with may change before they're a year old. Despite what many people say, not all babies are born with blue eyes, especially dark-skinned ones.

◎ Newborn babies often develop sucking blisters in the center of their top lip.

◎ The first poo, meconium, is like something out of a horror movie; thick and sticky, it looks like extruded, green-tinged tar, but once your milk "comes in" it gives way to the characteristic little-baby poo: yellowish and liquidy, with curds. This can come out at high velocity (kerrrrrr-SPLAT!), and you quickly learn to be ready at diaper change time to intercept a stream with the corner of a diaper. (And baby-boy pee can also travel quite a distance at short notice, in a large arc.)

◎ The early-baby pee may contain crystals that can make it look reddish. Disposable diapers have absorbent crystals that sometimes "escape" and look like tiny glass bubbles.

◎ The stump of the umbilical cord drops off in about a week or 2, and the hospital nurses will show you how to take care of it in the meantime.

◎ There is no medical reason for having baby boys circumcised, except in extremely rare cases. Some parents, however, insist on it for religious or cultural reasons. About 65 percent of newborn babies in the United States are circumcised each year. Circumcision is a very painful and shocking procedure for newborns when done without anesthesia. It's common for doctors to use local anesthesia and many doctors won't do the procedure without giving anesthesia. If a doctor is refusing to use anesthesia, the parents should find another, more progressive doctor. It's important to note that even with anesthesia the baby may experience some pain during the procedure and afterward. Expectant parents should research the pros and cons of having the procedure done before making a decision. Many religious parents are now leaving it to their son to make a decision about his own circumcision, when he comes of age and is able, unlike babies, to have a general anesthetic. You can check out the National Organization of Circumcision Information Resource Center's website (www.cirp.org) for information on choosing whether to circumcise your child. If you do choose circumcision, your obstetrician or pediatrician will generally perform the procedure.

your record

List of possible names:

Girl	Boy	Either

what's going on

The nesting urge is likely to be at fever pitch. Many women find themselves scrubbing underneath shelves and may have to be restrained. Don't do anything that involves standing on a chair or a ladder, no matter how much you feel that dusting the curtain rod is crucial to life as we know it. You might have aches and pains caused by your ginormous uterus. A gentle walk should help.

The baby is technically "full term"—that is, fully developed—as it enters this week, although most doctors say 40 weeks is full term too because that's the typical length of a pregnancy. Most of the lanugo has fallen out, but the baby's still covered in vernix. About a 1/2 ounce of fat is laid down each day from now on. The baby probably has a bowel full of meconium in a rather disgusting-looking hard rope of greeny-black stuff. Once the baby's out and starts on milk, the poo will be much more liquid. The baby still moves every day, but not very far. Weight: about 6 1/3 pounds.

DiARY Take Matt to see Dr. Herb, who says reassuring things about gigantic babies not necessarily being a problem because their moms' pelvises can handle it. Some of them simply pop out of their mothers singing a sea shanty, I'm sure. But he says he'll induce 10 days or so after the due date if I'm still lying around doing my walrus impressions. I inquire politely about which weekends he's not on call and promise to keep my legs crossed until he comes back on duty. The only time I can sleep properly is between 8 A.M. and noon. Luckily I don't have to be anywhere.

Because it's all a bit exhausting. Have taken to not returning phone calls and living in my robe. Wish I hadn't agreed to go into work once a week. Hard to exercise. Starting to think more about the baby coming home, and in deep denial about childbirth itself. (Surely it couldn't hurt that much. Maybe I could just buy a baby from a nice shop and avoid the whole thing.) I'm trying to focus on the advantage of having a big baby—it'll be more robust and less scary. Hang on a minute. All the advantages will come when it's out, and it's not out yet.

I try to think about what kind of person the baby will be, but get grumpy and tell Matt off for putting the wrong things in the fridge, when it was really me all the time and I'd forgotten and maybe this is some kind of weird pregnancy Jekyll and Hyde thing, or maybe it isn't and . . . Anyway, whatever. I'm all nested out. The house is getting untidy again, but I can't deal with cleaning it. At least I know that Matt will make the house spotless before I bring the baby home because otherwise he knows I would have him killed.

Even more drugstores have started thrusting sample bags at me full of pamphlets and tiny-sized stuff. Heartburn lozenges, diaper rash lotions, pads for bleeding, pads for incontinence (oh GOD), ads for safety seats and equipment, safety hats, safety pants, safety booties, lures to get you into Toys 'R' Us, and 400 different kinds of disposable diapers. They certainly give the impression that children are (a) dangerous and (b) moist.

info

your body after the birth

immediately afterward

After the birth of your baby, you might feel shivery and shaky, ecstatic, exhausted, sore, empty, blank, numb, sleepy, or wide awake: whatever you feel is okay, and certainly won't be unprecedented. (At least one woman has taken the first look at her baby and said, "Where did that come from?") If you've had an epidural, you may still have a pee catheter in your urethra and an IV drip in your hand.

Putting the baby to the breast as soon as possible after birth helps stimulate the uterus to contract and to squeeze out the placenta. Your new baby might not be hungry yet, but it's nice to meet a nipple anyway.

in the following days

Bleeding (lochia) The lochia—the discharge of blood, mucus and tissue from the uterus—will continue for 2 to 8 weeks after the birth. It is kind of like having a period at first, with some clots. It changes to a pink or brownish color and ends as a yellow-white discharge.

◉ Have on hand plenty of maternity pads. (Because the cervix takes a while to close and tampons can cause infection, you can't use them until your first real period after the birth, and that could be months away if you're breastfeeding.) You can use the new, ultra-absorbent, thin pads if you like, but the extra padding of the thicker supersize pads might make sitting more comfy.

◉ Tell your obstetrician if you have very heavy bleeding (soaking more than one pad an hour), the discharge has a yucky smell, or you have a fever. Also tell the obstetrician right away if you don't bleed at all in the days or weeks after giving birth.

"Afterpains" "Afterpains" usually occur for a few days or more after you have given birth, as your uterus contracts back toward its normal size. It's quite common to feel afterpains during breast-feeding.

Hemorrhoids and constipation

◉ Labor and delivery can give you hemorrhoids, a distension of the blood vessels at the entrance to your anus. Try not to strain when you poo, even if you're constipated, because it will make the hemorrhoids worse. Some people don't poo for a few days, especially after a cesarean, and you might need help from stool softeners. Ask your obstetrician for a prescription or recommendations for over-the-counter remedies.

◉ If you have hemorrhoids, ask your obstetrician, midwife, or the nursing staff about icepacks and ointment for relief.

◉ You may also need to eat more fruit, vegetables, and cereals for fiber, and drink lots of water. See the hints on how to avoid constipation in the info in Week 8.

Your poor sore vulva area There will usually be "some level of discomfort in the perineal area," as doctors say, after a vaginal delivery, ranging from bearable to excruciating; you may need some pain relief for a day or 2 after delivery. If you've had an episiotomy or tear, the nurses in the hospital will show you how to look after the stitched area so that it heals up well, and the site will be regularly checked for infection before you go home.

◎ Regular baths or sitz baths with salt or *very diluted* (10 drops per bath) tea-tree oil can help the healing process.

◎ Wash stitched areas gently, even just with water, two or three times a day.

◎ Dry the area well after bathing and give yourself some pants-off airing time if possible.

◎ Don't dry stitches with a hair dryer unless you have a cool setting—some people numb the area with ice or drugs and then scorch themselves with a hair dryer that's too hot or too close. It might be better to wave a paper fan or a handy copy of the *National Equirer*.

◎ If your stitches are sore and itchy, try dissolving a teaspoon of bicarbonate of soda or salt in warm water, then sitting in it after a pee.

◎ Try leaning forward (with your hands reaching toward the floor) when you pee so that pee doesn't get onto the stitches.

◎ Splash out (so to speak) on some thick, soft toilet paper.

◎ While having a poo in the first couple of days post-delivery, you might find it more comfortable if you support the perineal area firmly with a pad or wad of toilet paper.

◎ Avoid constipation by keeping your fiber intake up and drinking plenty of water.

◎ Don't sit on a rubber ring—it will direct more blood to the area, creating more pressure.

◎ Sit on a rolled-up towel or with a pillow under each buttock.

◎ Fill a condom with water and freeze it, and then wrap it in a washcloth and pop it in your panties.

◎ Ask your doctor to prescribe anti-inflammatories or pain killers that won't be transferred to the baby in breast milk.

◎ Take vitamin C for healing. Ask your naturopath or independent midwife for doses or follow instructions on the bottle.

◎ Pelvic-floor exercises will stimulate circulation in the area and assist in the healing process. The first few times the area will feel very tired and trembly, and you may have some numbness, but do as many as you can as soon as you can.

◎ Most doctors say no sex until the 6-week checkup at least— possibly *after* the 6-week checkup would be better (*during* might be considered a little inconsiderate).

◎ If you think you have a urinary tract infection, call your doctor right away.

your record

What are your feelings about breastfeeding?
Are you determined to do it? How long would you
like to breastfeed for? What if you can't?

SOME STRETCH MARK ZONES
(ARROWED)

EEK 39

what's going on

The cervix gets softer and thinner, ready to open wide enough for a baby's head to come through. Any time now it could release the mucous plug, which will end up on your underwear and is a sign that labor could start within hours or days. The uterus is practicing contractions; possibly confusing you about whether it's actually labor or not. You are probably completely fed up with being pregnant and have forgotten what your feet look like.

Your baby's genitals at this point have been overexcited by all your extra hormones and will be very large indeed in comparison to the rest of the body. They will return to a more seemly size a few days after the birth.

Weight: about 7 pounds.

Average approximate baby length this week from head to butt

Diary ─ Latest inventory of body changes: gigantic, veiny boozoombas with brown nipples; new, brown, flat moles on them, and heaps of skin tags under each one; huuuge tummy; purple, stripey stretch marks on boobs and hips. And I can't see my legs or pubic hair. For all I know they've been stolen.

I know why whales beach themselves. THEY JUST CAN'T BE BOTHERED ANY MORE.

Having a baby is a preposterous proposition. How can this huge, hard thing possibly come out of a vagina? I hear about a woman whose first words after labor were "What a completely shocking thing to happen." I've also heard so many stories about people looking blankly at their newborn baby and wondering what on earth to do with it. I'm determined not to panic if I don't bond right away.

I ask Marg, "Is it like an out-of-body experience?"

"No," she says. "It's a get-out-of-my-body experience."

I still can't tell what my body wants—am I hungry, tired, nauseous, getting a cold? I have no idea. Walking is hard now, the damn groin pain never goes away: those ligaments must be under so much strain the anchor points are constantly stressed.

The word "deliver" is sexist, says one pregnancy book, because it indicates a male doctor does the work of "delivery." That's crap. The mom's delivering—just like a FedEx van. How about "de-mommed," or would the mom be "de-babied"? One person has already asked if I have been "unsprogged."

At this week's visit, Dr. Herb looks exhausted—he's been up all night delivering babies. I didn't sleep much either.

"Is anything worrying you? Is there anything you want to ask?"

"No. Except don't go off duty, and did you get your motorcycle license?"

Turns out he didn't do it 2 weeks ago, so now he's going for the test this Saturday.

"I want to roar up next to some of the other doctors at the lights and see the looks on their faces," he says. (Apparently the other doctors were shocked when he shaved off his beard. They sound pretty easy to shock. Maybe he should just start cross-dressing.)

People are so different about babies. Attitudes range from the clucky to the disbelieving, through to distaste and secrecy.

I told my accountant, "I feel stupid and tired."

She was horrified I'd said it aloud. "Don't tell anyone!"

There is a conspiracy of working mothers to hide the effects of pregnancy and motherhood so as not to be discriminated against.

I look up "pregnant ladies" on the Internet and the first eleven matches are hardcore porn sites.

info

feeding your new baby

You may as well read this now because you won't feel like reading it right after your baby's born! It's hard to think past labor at the moment, but when it's over you'll be preoccupied with your breasts.

Breastfeeding is the best way to feed because breast milk is perfectly designed to nourish your baby with all the right nutrients and supply antibodies to boost the baby's immune system, which formula can't deliver.

BaBy's fAVORiTe VieW

In the past, babies were weaned onto plain old cow's milk, which wasn't very good for them, being designed for calves, not human babies, but now infant formulas are specially designed to give as many of the nutrients in breast milk as possible. Formula still runs second, but it's a much better second than it used to be.

breastfeeding in the first days

⊚ For the first few days after birth the baby will be drinking the creamy yellow premilk, colostrum, which is specially designed to nourish a baby and provide it with antibodies before it gets the milk. Most babies will lose a bit of weight until the milk "comes in," and then start to gain again.

◎ At first breastfeeding might be painful, especially if your baby is having trouble latching on properly (latching on is often called "attachment") and chomps on the nipple or can't seem to stay on and suck. The baby needs to take most of the areola as well as the nipple in its mouth and the nipple goes to the back of the mouth. Different mothers and babies find different feeding positions suit them best. Use your time in the hospital to get as much help and advice from the staff as you need.

◎ If you're having problems breastfeeding and feel that the hospital staff have done all they can to help you, or they don't have the time, or they are giving you conflicting advice, ask them to get the hospital's lactation consultant, or a private consultant, to come and see you.

◎ When your milk comes in (usually after 3 or 4 days), you can expect your breasts to feel full and hard. The staff or your own midwife will be able to give you advice on how to ease this, such as expressing a little milk before each feed and applying hot washcloths or cabbage leaves. You might need a cream to keep them supple: lactation consultants most often recommend pure lanolin. You don't need "tough" nipples, you want pliable ones.

◎ You might be asked if you can feel your milk "coming in." This is like a shiver, a tingling, a prickle or even a stabbing pain in each breast, though sometimes you don't feel it for days or even weeks after the birth—or ever—but the "let down" of your milk will be happening before or during each and every breastfeed.

◎ If you can, try to let your nipples air dry after feeding. Exposing them to very mild sunlight for short periods (3–5 minutes) will dry any excess moisture, and the ultraviolet light helps them to heal.

hooray for boobs

Because breast milk is so fabulous for babies, because it helps you to bond with your baby, and because it's on tap and free of charge, it's really worth persevering even if you have initial trouble breast-feeding: very few babies and mothers can get their act together right away. The thing to remember is to try to relax (I know it's hard at the time when you've got a hungry, crying baby and you can't get it to "attach" properly). Take a deep breath and lower your shoulders. It takes time for you and the baby to learn breast-feeding together. A middle road could be expressing your milk occasionally and putting it in a bottle to give your nipples a rest. You can also supplement a low supply with formula. Even managing 6 days or 6 weeks of breastfeeding is a big bonus for your baby. And if it really doesn't work, you have a fine backup with formula: your baby will not starve. So give it another try.

Quite often you'll get conflicting advice from hospital nurses about how to hold the baby and how to position yourself while you feed. If it's all putting your head in a whirl (you'll be madly sleep deprived, which doesn't help), choose to listen to ONE of them—call in the lactation consultant, for example, and don't be swayed from their advice if it's working. Choose someone who clearly likes babies, is encouraging and gentle, and takes the time to help you, sit with you, watch your technique, and try different ways to help. (Don't choose anyone who grabs your breast in one hand, the baby in the other, and brings them together like a clash of cymbals.)

La Leche League has trillions of booklets, pamphlets, videos, and books available to help you solve a bewildering array of breastfeeding problems and can be a marvelous support. I suspect if you want to breastfeed a Down's syndrome baby upside down in an igloo, there'll be a pamphlet on it.

Ask for practical advice, not just encouragement to continue breastfeeding. Some associations may be able to encourage you but may not have the special skills to help. Even if your breastfeeding is not well-established when you leave the hospital, there are lactation outpatient practices, lactation specialists who will do home visits, and pediatric offices with lactation experts available to help.

You may find that in their zeal for breastfeeding, some people gloss over the real problems you're having, with the advice "Just keep trying." If you think breastfeeding is "taking too much out of you," it probably is—don't accept that this is "nonsense" or inevitable: get some nutritional and coping advice. If you're finding it impossible to juggle work and breastfeeding, don't just accept that "Many other women do it and you can too": make sure you get practical help on how to continue.

 For more info, see Breastfeeding in Help.

not breastfeeding

If the worst comes to the worst and you can't breastfeed your baby or breastfeeding is not for you, it's nowhere near the end of the world. The way people go on about it, you'd think not breastfeeding was the equivalent of making the baby drink gin and wheeling it across freeways during blizzards in a war zone. Plenty of bottle-fed babies grow up to be strapping, robust, healthy adults. Look at the adults around you. Look at the kids around you. Can you tell who was bottle-fed? 'Course you can't. Many other factors affect a child's development and immune system, including the amount of chemicals in an environment, access to fresh and healthy food, and exposure and building up a resistance to germs.

It would be lovely if you could breastfeed, but you can't. Instead you can enjoy the relaxed feeling of bottle-feeding your baby while making eye contact, and the freedom it gives you because you can always get somebody else to feed the baby if you'd like to go out for an hour or so and have an affair with a couple of firemen. Now tweak those two nipples—not those, the ones that fit on the bottle. And get on with it.

Your pediatrician can help you with all the stuff you need to know about sterilizing equipment and storing and heating bottles.

Stuff to tell nosy people
"I have an illness controlled by medication, which mustn't be passed through breast milk to my baby."

"Both my nipples blew off during a wind storm."

"I have an antibiotic-resistant form of infected breasts, and either of them could explode at any moment."

"It's easier to get the gin into a bottle."

"Both my boobs were removed years ago."

"I can't breastfeed, and I don't want to talk about it. Gosh, that's a lovely blouse."

"So far five lactation specialists have told me I'm one of those women who just can't breastfeed. In the old days I would have had a wet nurse."

"Oh, just PISS OFF."

what's going on This is the magic week when your baby is "due," unless somebody has messed up the dates. But this is based on averages, so don't expect to give birth on the due date. If you do, it is simply showing off.

The baby is rounder and fatter and probably ready to be born. It is now about 200 times heavier than it was at twelve weeks. Boys are often bigger than girls. Weight: about 7$\frac{1}{2}$ pounds.

WEEK 40

DiARY

I'm due. And I am nothing but a limbo-living, dimply-assed, stoned giantess. When I go to see Dr. Herb the women in the waiting room who are only a couple of months pregnant look at me with very contemplative expressions: "Surely I couldn't get THAT big," I hear them saying in their innermost thoughts.

Matt has suggested we change the name of the baby to Godot, and I am like a cat waiting to have kittens, prowling around the house looking for a good cupboard to give birth in—or tidy up. I'm finding it harder to drink Beck's herbal uterine tonic concoction—I'm just sick of it, but I persevere because she says I have good uterine tone, which I am immensely proud of, it being the only part of my body that HAS ANY TONE.

Obsessed with the idea of labor. Someone reminds me of Kathy Lette's description of a post-cesarean vagina as "honeymoon fresh." If I didn't laugh I'd sob m'self silly. It's also becoming clear to me how many pregnant women worry about pooing during labor. I'm just surprised your lungs don't come out your butt considering all the pressure.

Have left a message on the answering machine saying nothing's happened yet. People calling and asking all the time. All the ones who are already mothers say, "Good luck," "Take the drugs," and "You're not going to try and have a natural birth are you?"

Uncle Stan turns up on the doorstep dressed like a Hollywood B-movie costume designer's idea of a part-time pimp: opaque, yellow-lensed, concave, wraparound sunglasses; ankle-length leather jacket; high-heeled boots; and gray beard. I try not to stare. Aurelia is always waiting in the car, usually taking advantage of the mirror on the inside of the passenger sun shade.

He hands me a sack of organic lentils and remarks casually that he and Aurelia are going on vacation next week to a commune.

"So," I venture, "you won't be here when the baby's born?"

"Leave a message on the answering machine!" he cries gaily as he heads for the gate.

Family support. What would you do without it? Get along all right, is my guess.

My dream birth: I am lying on a sexy, dusky pink satin-quilted four-poster bed reading a magazine full of photos of gorgeous clothes I could afford that would look quite nice on me (I *said* it was a dream) when a man in a leopard-skin suit comes past with a cocktail cart on wheels full of excellent cakes, bottles of attractively colored alcohol, an ice bucket, and some syringes.

"Martini?" he inquires politely. "Or would madam care for an epidural?"

Just at that moment a perfectly charming baby pops out of my vagina.

"Ow," I remark, absentmindedly. "Why, thank you, I'll take a gin and lime. And a small colostrum for my new young friend."

Just in case this doesn't happen, Dr. Herb has scheduled me to go into the maternity hospital next Monday at 5 P.M. to have my cervix annointed with a prostaglandin that mimics the one in the body that basically says, "Lady, start your engines for labor." I have to stay in the hospital, and they might put some more in the next morning. Then I might be able to start on my own without the pitocin drip, although in most cases an IV pitocin drip would be started and the membranes have to be broken by the doctor if the waters don't break by themselves. This is scary.

Had a problem sleeping last night, thinking about bringing a baby home, and cesarean, and pain . . .

Beck's given me acupuncture twice to try to move the baby along a bit, and I've taken some tiny homeopathic pills. The baby finally "engages" (goes into firing position) after 2 days of this. So TIRED. Some anxiety attacks, but mostly sort of numb.

Everyone is calling up saying, "Has anything happened?"

"NO!"

info

your hospital stay

Staff nurses will be assigned to you in the hospital. Their job is to take care of you as you recover from the birth. They are also there to help you learn how to feed and look after your baby. Ask them anything you want to know, and take full advantage of their time and knowledge. Most women spend 1 to 3 days in the hospital after giving birth, and often 3 to 5 after a cesarean. You can ask to be discharged when you feel ready to go home, providing you and your baby get the all clear from medical staff. If you do go home early, a visit to the pediatrician is encouraged soon after you are home.

exercise

If your hospital or gym offers postnatal exercise or physical therapy classes, try to go. It's a good way to get into an exercise routine that you will hopefully continue in the weeks after you get home, it will help your body recover, and moving about should help you to feel less stiff and sore. (Actually you probably won't have the time or energy for exercises for a while. If you do, that's great. If you don't, don't beat yourself up about it. But do go to the classes so that when you get a minute, you'll know what to do.)

food

◎ Nutrition and beating hunger are important issues for breast-feeding. Ask your lactation consultant, hospital dietician, independent midwife, or naturopath for suggestions.

◎ It may be nutritionally sound, but hospital food is usually, at best, pathetically boring. Get friends to bring you decent food such as fresh fruit. Most wards have a fridge and access to a micro-wave so you can have a stash of your own.

visitors

◉ Don't feel obliged to see everyone who wants to check out the baby while you're in the hospital. Make the most of this time when your meals, cleaning, and other needs are being taken care of by other people to recover from the birth and to prepare yourself for when you go home. If you like, ban all but a few close friends and family from visiting for the first few days so you can rest and spend time with your baby.

◉ Visiting hours are not as strict as they used to be, but you can pretend that they are, or choose a hospital where they are. If you don't want people dropping in outside the set hours, enlist the help of the nurses and ward staff.

◉ If you have a phone, you can ask the switchboard to take messages for you so that you can call out but the phone doesn't ring all the time.

⊚ Ask people to phone you before they come to visit. If you're too tired or don't feel up to seeing anyone, you can ask them to come another time.

⊚ If flowers get in the way and cause allergies, ask people who are coming to visit you not to bring them. Instead have one or two close friends bring you a small bunch to brighten things up.

paperwork and other nitty-gritties

Birth notice You might want to write a paragraph for the news-paper's birth announcements and keep that edition for the baby when they grow up.

Registering the birth This should be done as soon as possible after the birth, once you've got the name sorted out. Birth certificates are created for infants at the hospital right after birth. Usually the staff will provide you with a worksheet to complete the birth certificate, and you will sign the original. The original will be forwarded to county offices, from which you can order a copy. You also have the option to apply for a Social Security number for your baby by filling out some extra paperwork.

If you're not sure what involvement the father wants with the child, or the father isn't around, get legal advice from a com-munity legal center or your own lawyer about whether to put his name on the certificate. It's quite okay to leave the father bit blank if you need to. Don't let anyone write "unknown" or anything judgmental for the kid to read when they grow up and get a copy. If you're not happy with the birth certificate, you can have it altered.

Health insurance coverage If you have health insurance, check with your human resources department or insurance company about adding your baby to the policy. Usually this needs to happen within 30 days of the birth, or the baby's hospital bill after the birth may not be covered. If you do not have insurance, you may qualify for government-funded Medicaid provided your income is low enough. Medicaid covers any service deemed "medically necessary" for you and your baby. If you do not qualify for Medicaid because your income is over the limit, but you can't afford insurance, check with your state's Children's Health Insurance Program (CHIP). CHIP provides for checkups, immunizations, doctor's visits, prescription costs, eyeglasses, and hospital care for uninsured children.

what's going on

If your pregnancy has been "average" (40 weeks long), your baby is out in the world and perhaps sleeping off the shock. After your baby is born a whole bunch of hormonal activities happen, quite suddenly. Your body expels the placenta, which has been pumping out huge quantities of hormones. Suddenly you're bereft of the "happy hormones" and getting a boost of hormones such as prolactin to help breastfeeding. Your body looks less pregnant, but your tummy is still very big. You're bleeding from the vagina as the body expels all that nice uterine surface the baby needed. Your body is recovering from the massive shock of childbirth—whether vaginal or surgical. Give yourself a break. Don't do anything but recover and be with your baby.

The baby may have some characteristic newborn marks, such as "stork bites" (red, rashlike shapes on the forehead, eyelids, and/or back of the neck) or temporary marks from forceps. More than half of all newborn babies develop a temporary yellowy tinge to the skin and eyeballs, called jaundice—it's usually no big deal. Your baby is sucking colostrum because your milk probably won't come in until day 3 or 4. The bub will be down a bit from its birth weight before the breast milk kicks in. Don't worry about this: too much scientific measuring and talk of weight-loss percentages can be freaky—lost weight in those first few days is expected in all babies and the loss can be made up in just a few days.

WEEK 41

pleased to meet you

DiARY

It's time. We drive to the hospital, with the bag neatly packed with all the things we'll need for labor, to meet Herb for the prostaglandin induction, feeling nervous but excited. Luckily Maternity isn't busy so we get our own room with a big hospital bed, which Matt bounces on. Sleep! Can't imagine it myself.

In the morning, when contractions will probably start, I'll call Beck and tell her to come in sporting her best midwifery hat.

Dr. Herb comes into our room wearing a lovely suit and some Calvin Klein aftershave on his way to a movie premiere with his wife, and puts the gel in my vagina. What a charming bedside manner he has—he chats away about something else and one could almost be at a dinner party if he didn't have his hand up your vagina.

A nice Lorraine-y nurse arrives in a white jacket and navy pants and puts a piece of electronic equipment on wheels next to the bed and attaches a belt around my tummy. This is the monitor. It continually rolls out a graph of any contractions and a graph of the baby's heartbeat, which is usually up around 150 beats a minute. Matt and I start to play cards, pretending that we can keep our mind on gin rummy instead of all the machinery.

A long time later I write this: Suddenly I noticed that the baby's heartbeat had dropped to 80 beats a minute and the graph line was plunging down like a sheer cliff face. And so began the worst 2 hours of my life.

Matt tried to reassure me that it was probably normal, but when the nurse came back she got a look on her face I never want to see again and called Dr. Herb, who, it transpires, was just reaching for his first foie gras hors d'oeuvre at the film premiere. Within 15 minutes he was back in the room, looking at the graph.

"I'm just going outside to consult with someone, and I'll be back in a moment to tell you what we're going to do," he said calmly.

Left alone, Matt and I held hands and tried not to look as frightened as the other.

"He's going to do an emergency cesarean. I guess Beck's not going to make it in time," I thought suddenly.

Herb came back in and sat on the bed, and held my hand and said—oh dear, I still can't write these words without crying—

"Your baby is distressed, and if it's this distressed because of a small contraction, we won't risk going through labor."

Behind the scenes an anesthesiologist, a pediatrician, and another obstetrician were rushing in from their homes or elsewhere in the building. They took Matt away, which was awful, and they quickly wheeled me out on one of those cold, gleaming carts and into the white, shining operating room, where there were people with blue paper masks, shower caps, and gowns. ("Nice to see some fashion coordination," I thought, ages later. At the time I wasn't thinking much at all. I was just frightened.)

The anesthesiologist put an IV drip in my left hand and then gave me a spinal-block injection into the lower back, with me curled in a fetal position while a nurse held my hand. It was really scary staying perfectly still so he didn't get the wrong bit of the spine. As the anesthetic started to work, Dr. Herb came back in with the nurse, a pediatrician, the other obstetrician, and—thank God!—Matt, who looked like he was playing an extra in *ER*. They put up a blue fabric screen over my chest so I couldn't see my tummy. Everyone fussed around behind the screen for a moment.

"Let me know when you start," I said to Dr. Herb.

Everybody laughed.

"We've been in for 3 minutes," he said.

When I looked up at the huge light with the flat globe cover, I could see the reflection of my insides, yellow and pink and purple. These were the things I was thinking: "Please let my baby be all right," "Thank God I live in a First World country," "Thank God I'm not having a home birth," and large stretches of blank that probably had something to do with shock.

"There's your baby coming out," said one of the nurses, taking a Polaroid photo.

"Is it Eddy or Pearl?" I asked.

"It's Eddy!" everyone chorused.

And suddenly Herb held up a silent, purple, slimy creature with a screwed up, tiny little face and a smudge of dark hair. A sob caught in my throat as I reached out and gently touched my baby's leg with the back of my hand. I didn't know if any other contact would hurt Eddy or be the wrong thing to do.

Instantly he was whipped away to a table by the pediatrician and the nurse, who started to check everything.

"He's got all the right things in all the right places," said the pediatrician.

And then Eddy started to cry. All the experienced people in the room broke into huge smiles.

"That's a good cry," they said simultaneously, and you could feel the relief in the room.

The two obstetricians were doing their downstairs needlework on what Matt would later refer to as "the tummy smile": my curved red scar. The pediatrician, the nurse, and Matt whisked out to go and do tests on Eddy. For some reason I told Matt through my tears—I couldn't stop crying—not to let Eddy out of his sight. (As if he was going to duck out to the bar for a few cold ones.) The obstetricians finished and went away, and two nurses wheeled me next door into the recovery room and gave me a lemonade popsicle, and there I stayed for about an hour, drugged out of my mind and not really believing it had happened, and wondering where my baby was.

When finally I was wheeled back into our room, there were Matt and Eddy. I was really worried that Eddy was all right, but I didn't feel an immediate surge of overwhelming love. Mostly relief that he was okay, and confusion about how to get him on the breast for a snack of colostrum. Eddy just looked tired and tiny, and slept a lot. And guess what? He wasn't even a whopper: 7 pounds 13 ounces. Damn. All the rest was Haagen Dazs.

info

coping when you get home

getting organized

ⓖ To stop people dropping in at all hours, insist that friends and relatives call before visiting or set aside particular times (say, certain mornings a week).

ⓖ If friends or relatives offer to help with cleaning, cooking, or shopping, ACCEPT IMMEDIATELY!

ⓖ There will be days when preparing dinner will seem impossible or unbearable. Prepare for these by cooking extra, large batches when you make things that can be frozen such as soups and casseroles. If friends and relations offer to bring you meals, ACCEPT IMMEDIATELY! Keep take-out menus from a few decent local places.

ⓖ Ask friends to chip in to hire a cleaner for the first month or so instead of giving you flowers and fancy baby accessories. Instead of lots of outfits, ask a couple of friends to buy bibs. You'll soon find out why: much easier to whip on and off than change a whole sticky outfit.

ⓖ If you can afford it, get a cleaning service in for a few hours every 1 or 2 weeks so that the basic housework, such as cleaning the bathroom and kitchen, is always done.

ⓖ If you can't afford a cleaning service but can't stand being in a messy house, just keep one room tidy. This will give you somewhere to relax or see visitors.

ⓖ If you live by yourself, try to organize a roster of friends to come by each day for the first few weeks so that you can have an uninterrupted half hour to take a shower or bath, sit down without the baby, or get out of the house briefly.

looking after yourself

⑥ Ask someone you trust to look after your baby while you do something relaxing such as going for a walk or seeing a friend.

⑥ Try to get out of the house every day to help keep yourself sane. If you're going somewhere like a shopping center, check out the parents' facilities and whether there are elevators or escalators. If you have to negotiate a lot of stairs, you may be better off with a baby front pack than a stroller.

⑥ Try to get time each day to do your postnatal exercises (especially the pelvic-floor ones)—you'll find you have more energy for them in the mornings. If you enjoy exercising with other people, a postnatal class after a few weeks will also give you a chance to talk with other new mothers.

⑥ If you have a partner, make time to go out alone with them, even if it's just for coffee.

⑥ Make sure your partner understands that most women don't feel like flinging themselves into chandelier-swingin' rumpy pumpy for a few weeks at least. It might be nice to break this more gently than placing a sign saying "Off Limits" over your crotch.

⑥ Use the time when your baby is sleeping during the day to have a nap or relax. Put your needs ahead of visitors, housework, and other chores.

⑥ Don't pretend you're coping if you're not: share things with your partner or friends.

⑥ If you feel you need more help than you can get at home, ask your doctor to refer you to a program that helps with parenting skills, like feeding, settling, and looking after your baby.

a crying baby

Small babies often cry for mysterious reasons. Here are some tips to stop your baby crying if they are not hungry, tired, hot, cold, wet, or in pain from gas or a diaper pin or whatever else you've checked for:

⑥ curl up together in bed in a warm, dark, quiet room, tummy to tummy for maximum skin contact.

⑥ try a warm (not hot) bath and baby massage (some babies hate both until they're a few weeks old)—ask a nurse for a demo; basically, be gentle, use any sort of oil you can eat, and stop if it makes the baby cranky.

⑥ rock with your baby in a chair.

⑥ play soothing music (you might feel like a dope but sing to your baby— anything soothing, even if you have to make it up—and if you "can't sing," your baby won't notice).

⑥ walk with a gentle rhythmic bounce or sway in your step up and down a hall about 5,000 times with the baby over your shoulder.

⑥ try to distract the baby by holding them level with your face and nodding your head, while making a (pleasant) noise or grinning—this can give them such a surprise that they forget what they were crying about.

⑥ go about your business with the baby in a front pack.

⑥ try a pacifier approved for newborns.

⑥ accept there's nothing you can do, and get someone else in to hold the baby while you walk around the block.

For more info, see Crying and Parent Services in Help.

getting your baby to sleep

◉ Ask your hospital nurses how you can recognize when to put your baby down to sleep, and if you need a "routine."

◉ Try to get into a settling routine when your baby is due to go down so that they start to associate certain things with relaxing and going to sleep. You might use sounds (singing, music, or even rhythmic noises like the washing machine), movements such as rocking in a chair or baby swing or being carried close to your body in a baby pouch, massage, a ride in a stroller or car, or a warm bath. (A car is an expensive habit to get into and not great if you're exhausted.)

◉ Use a dimmer switch or soft lamp to feed by at nighttime, and avoid talking to or stimulating the baby or they'll think it's play time.

◉ Overtiredness is a common cause of crying, which paradoxically can make it harder for the baby to get to sleep. A baby can seem "hyped up" when they're really overtired. Soothing methods that involve walking, rocking, or singing to the baby may end up stimulating them more, so that it is harder to get them to sleep. Instead, try stroking your baby's head or tummy, patting your baby's back rhythmically, or make soothing hushing sounds.

◉ You don't need to be silent while your baby is sleeping. It's best for them to get used to normal noise levels, or you'll always have to have a silent house.

and the rest
For all the other stuff you'll worry about such as gas, vomiting, and weird-lookin' poo, see your doctor, peruse Help, and always have a baby-care book on hand (see Baby-Care Books in Week 43).

 For more info, see Sleeping and Parent Services in Help.

your record

Scribble down everything about your labor. I know
you don't believe it now, but you will forget!

YOUR UTERUS IS SHRINKING

what's going on

Your uterus is slowly shrinking, contracting each time you breastfeed, it will be back to its right size in about 6 weeks. Your muscles and ligaments are all adjusting to the loss of relaxin. Retained fluid may still cause puffy ankles and sore joints, especially the knees, and the problem may stick around for some weeks.

Your baby will be starting to grow at a very fast rate. Sometimes it will seem as if you can see the difference in a day. Your baby can't see very much, because their eyes only focus on things within 10 inches, and probably isn't smiling yet: this can make a baby seem very passive and not much fun. But before you know it they'll be staring at you with eyes on full-beam, and within about 5 weeks you'll be seeing gorgeous gummy grins.

WEEK 42

Diary

I'm writing all this down later, as the week after Eddy's birth was a hideous haze of drug-addled fatigue and incomprehension. I know I'm supposed to say it was a wonderful, joyous time full of relief and the tinkling laughter of well-dressed parents overwhelmed with a sense of achievement, and that sort of palaver, but it was a damned nightmare.

Poor old Eddy, the least experienced of us all in the ways of the world, was plonked into a room with two sleep-deprived, deeply gobsmacked parents, one of whom was on drugs and a bed on wheels, wired up to a drip and in pain, and the other of whom didn't have any breasts. Not that we weren't happy to see Eddy. But I kept looking at him through a veil of painkillers that seemed to deaden brain feelings as well as pain.

I just couldn't connect Eddy with who used to be inside me, especially because he had been taken away when he was born and I lay there outside the operating room for all that time in a surreal state—not pregnant, but without a baby. At first he just didn't feel like mine—maybe it was because we hadn't gone on the journey of labor together, and I hadn't felt him being born. Maybe it was because of the drugs or the shock, or because having a real live baby actually felt hyper-real.

Eddy looked exactly like Matt without the 5 o'clock shadow. He had a very serious expression, and fists that could be gently opened into small starfish and mother-of-pearl fingernails. He was so tiny and lovable, and so mysterious and passive. It felt like we were constantly doing things TO him—trying to breastfeed him, changing diapers, wrapping and unwrapping him. His vulnerable "littleness" made me feel very protective and scared at the same time.

Matt was in shock for days afterward, I think. He kept trying to make everyone cups of tea and explain soccer to a very deadpan Eddy. We spent ages looking at Eddy's little face, wondering what he was thinking. "Probably 'get me another bosom,'" said Matt.

The daytime nurses were mostly wonderful, especially the ones who would change the sheets and help tidy up the room. If I had to do it over again, I would have asked Aunt Peg or Jill or someone to help every day—it's just not something you can usually do yourself, especially after major surgery.

Eddy's bed was a plastic tub on a cart that they'd take away to the nursery at night when I got completely exhausted. And then the night nurses—oh my God, the night nurses. Two were brilliant. The rest were more trouble than they were worth. I got to dread pressing the button for help at night because a nurse would bustle or burst in, cross from being drawn away from the nursery, or just cross.

They would gruffly grab Eddy with one hand and my breast with the other and bring them together with the force of somebody applauding heartily. After this tense-making and confronting behavior, often accompanied by barked instructions, they would push down on my shoulders and command, "Relax! You're supposed to enjoy it!" or pull me into a position a previous nurse had insisted was completely wrong.

One night nurse was so bad we held our breath when she came into the room. Literally bursting through the door like Cranky Bart in a bad Western movie, she stomped across to turn off the call button and jabbed her finger at the wall so hard she injured herself.

Shaking her finger and glowering, she stood over us and asked, "What do you want?"

"My painkiller was due an hour ago," I said.

She reached into her pocket for the tablet, slapped it into my palm, and stomped off again. "Just call if you need anything," she snarled, and slammed the door.

Yeah, right. Maybe if I were on FIRE.

One night I went up to the nursery to get Ed back and I could hear him crying. I looked at this little sobbing creature in one of the bassinets they use to settle babies, and leaned in and cradled the baby to me. The crying stopped immediately and I cuddled and soothed for a moment, then turning to take him back to my room I happened to notice from the wristband that I had picked up the baby of Rabbi Fierstein and his lovely wife, Rachel.

I turned to a midwife who had come over to see what I was doing. "Oh my God, I've got the wrong baby," I said.

"Yes." She smiled at me as if I were a complete maniac.

I slunk into the other nursery room where Eddy was happily listening to a lullaby and whisked him off to my room, feeling like an idiot, and an unfit mother who couldn't even recognize her own baby. No wonder all the babies have name tags attached.

I'm pretty sure it was the Rabbi and Rachel, dressed in full Orthodox gear, who met Matt in the corridor one morning and were rather arrested by the sight of Matt's gigantic pajamas covered in a cheerful print of rubber ducks. Matt's hair was sticking out to the side as if he were in a stiff wind, and the ear piece of one side of his glasses had snapped off, giving them a rather jaunty, 45-degree slant.

"Wow," said Matt.

Rachel averted her gaze, and the Rabbi just nodded as if something he had long suspected had been confirmed.

After about 3 or 4 days of Eddy waking up to be breastfed every 4 hours, a feeding that would take about an hour or more each time, I hadn't had more than 2 hours or so of sleep in a row. And for a person who needs 9 or 10 hours sleep a day, this was taking its toll. I did what I always do when I'm tired. I cried and cried.

It just felt like I couldn't cope, couldn't function with the immobility and pain and feeding the baby, if I didn't get some proper sleep. If they took Ed away to the nursery, they would bring him back when he was really hungry and screaming his head off— so he would be all worked up and unsettled and harder to feed and full of gas afterward, which meant more crying.

Anyway, it all culminated in me weeping uncontrollably after a bumbling attempt to feed Eddy with razor-painful nipples (one had a crack nobody could see except me) and watching a couple of nurses taking my baby away and telling me to sleep as they closed the door of my room behind them. I was almost hysterical thinking, "What's the point of sleeping? It will only be 2½ hours at the most! I may as well stay awake and go crazy."

And then I said to Matt, "They're all standing outside my room saying I can't cope and I've got postpartum depression. It's not the blues, I'm just overtired!" (Not to mention a touch paranoid.)

Well, they sent for a private lactation consultant, who turned up looking starched and sympathetic, and I decided if I was paying this woman for a consultation I would just listen to her advice and ignore any conflicting info from each shift of nurses. (By this time I was wearing a rather snug maternity bra as my boobs kept swelling up like cantaloupes.)

This turned out to be the best move to make because it meant I could continue to call her up for help when I got home from hospital. AND what's more, she could see the nipple crack. Well, she said she could.

So many people are rushed out of the hospital even before their milk comes in properly, and get into trouble when they arrive home with nobody to help. As far as breastfeeding goes, the only advice that you ever get is people saying "persevere," in different ways—this doesn't always help if you don't know HOW to persevere.

I called Beck nearly every day I was in the hospital (5 days) to tell her how tired and incompetent I felt. She sent in vitamin B, herbal tonics, and stern instructions to get out into the fresh air.

Eddy just lay wrapped up in a blanket looking at everything as if he were trying to memorize it. "Well, my friend," I said to him, "I'm sure I'll get better at this caper." Eddy presumably was thinking, "I'd like some more of that nipple business, if it's all the same to you, Leaky."

info

postpartum depression

what is it?

Most women experience what is known as the "baby blues"—feeling weepy and sad—often on about day 4 after giving birth when the "happy hormones" go and the prolactin kicks in for real milk production. For most women

wahwahwah
wahwahwah
wahwahwah

these blues only last a few days, but some find that the depression stays, or returns, and gets worse. It's hard to decide where the baby blues end and postpartum depression (PPD) begins, so figures for new mothers experiencing PPD vary from one in ten to more than half of all new moms. Recently there has been some research into the incidence of PPD in the partners of new mothers, with early findings suggesting that it could affect some men in the same way.

what causes it?
No one knows why PPD affects some women more than others, but hormones seem to be the main culprits. Estrogen and progesterone levels drop rapidly after childbirth, which may trigger depression in a way that is similar to fluctuating hormone levels causing PMS (premenstrual syndrome).

The following are all recognized as contributing factors in PPD and logical reasons why you may feel down:

◎ exhaustion—childbirth wears you out; so do visitors and trying to follow any kind of schedule once you have a baby. One of the reasons for exhaustion is that your volume of blood has suddenly been cut by 30 percent so a lesser volume is reaching your muscles than they have become used to, making them tire easily and feel weak. It takes a few weeks for your body to readjust to this. Sleep is one of the first things to suffer once the baby is born, and if you are depressed you can suffer from insomnia so you're unable to take advantage of even the ludicrously short sleep periods available to you.

◎ a traumatic birth—this can cause shock and disappointment.

◎ frustrating or bad hospital experiences—you might feel you need to get away from all the prodding, the unfamiliar cramped surroundings, and the artificial air.

◎ anxiety about coping—going home can seem overwhelming and terrifying when you think about how much you have to do, especially if you have other children to look after.

⊚ a sense of failure—this can arise from feeling unable to cope with all the things you think you "have" to do to be a good mother, disappointment if the birth didn't go according to plan, or feeling that you have somehow failed as a woman if you are having problems feeding and settling your baby. In reality, almost EVERYONE has a problem at some point.

⊚ a health problem—most new mothers will suffer from at least one following the birth: backache, fatigue, mastitis (infection of the milk ducts), painful episiotomy stitches, massive sleep deprivation. Feeling physically unwell adds to depression.

⊚ ennui—after spending 9 months on the high of anticipating seeing your baby for the first time, you may find yourself feeling underwhelmed. It is quite common to think that your baby is less than gorgeous or scintillating company until you have had time to bond emotionally. Tiny, new babies are very passive—there's none of the cooing, extended eye contact, and sticking their heads up out of flower pots we associate with babies (and greeting cards) for a few weeks or months yet. The guilt you experience when you feel bored by or distant from your baby only adds to the depression.

⊚ loss of individual identity—before the birth, everyone is focused on the pregnant woman and how she is feeling, and afterward many women feel that they are less important to their family and friends as all attention is on the baby. You may feel as if people have stopped seeing you as an individual and now see you only as a "mother."

⊚ perfectionist or anxious approach to life—PPD appears more in people who tend to worry or are perfectionists. Many women feel disappointed in themselves if they have always dealt with things to exacting standards in their professional and social lives and suddenly feel unable to reach that level of "perfection" in motherhood.

⊚ subsequent pregnancies—PPD is more common in women who already have children. Having to look after older children as well as a new baby is likely to place even tighter constraints on the time you have to yourself and to get enough rest. It can be scary wondering how you'll cope.

⑥ loneliness—if everyone you know is busy with their own lives and yours revolves around the baby, you may feel as though you are missing out on "life."

⑥ a feeling of being trapped in this lifestyle for the rest of your days—"Why on earth did I have a baby?"

Signs and symptoms:

⑥ the blues and the feelings listed above persist for more than a couple of weeks.

⑥ sleeplessness and/or lack of appetite.

⑥ low self-esteem.

⑥ confusion and/or panic attacks.

⑥ sadness.

⑥ feeling "flat."

⑥ feeling angry or aggressive toward yourself or your baby.

⑥ feeling desperately in over your head.

strategies

⑥ Set up a support network of family, friends, and professionals—accept help from others rather than feeling as if you have to prove you're capable by doing it all yourself. Remember that in sensible cultures babies are looked after by an extended family or even a whole tribe of people from the moment they're born. We weren't meant to do it alone.

⑥ Look after yourself—use the time when your baby sleeps to rest instead of catching up on all the things you think you should have done such as the housework; treat yourself to things that help you feel pampered and relaxed, such as a massage or haircut.

🌀 Get some fresh air—gentle exercise such as walking or yoga, with or without the baby, is calming and releases energy. Try to spend a little time each day realizing it IS day, and not just sleeping, eating, and feeding the baby in a twilight, indoor world.

🌀 Get together with other new moms—contact the women in your childbirth class or join a postpartum exercise class; or look online to figure out what times a new-mothers' group meets in your area: this will give you a chance to talk with women experiencing the same things and will help you feel part of something, rather than excluded.

🌀 If you think you may have PPD, ask your doctor to refer you to a therapist or counselor trained in PPD, and/or consider medications that are safe during breastfeeding. Lots of people find this really sorts them out.

🌀 Be aware that your partner, if you have one, might also have the blues. They might benefit from counseling or special help as well, and it's a good step for the baby's sake too.

 For more info, see Postpartum Depression in Help.

your record

Write down your first impressions of your baby:
whom the baby resembles, coloring, characteristics,
temperament, whatever.

How are you feeling ___ weeks in ?

Hospital/home visitors	Presents or flowers

what's going on

You're tired. You're still trying to get breastfeeding to be smooth and easy for both of you. Your body has started to heal. You're trying to cope with visitors as well as looking after the baby. You're in a dream world. FORGET THE DAMN HOUSEWORK.

You'll find that the tiny outfits that fitted in the first week start to get too small (the baby's outfits, not yours). Your baby's eye color may be changing, and the baby hair might be falling out, to be slowly replaced by a new lot. After another couple of weeks the shrivelled, stumpy bit of umbilical cord will come away from the navel and you'll see what your baby's belly button looks like. The hands will stay curled in fists for a few weeks yet. Length and weight? Oh who cares. Forget the statistics' for a minute. Every day your baby's getting closer to becoming a social being who sleeps more and doesn't cry so much (although the amount of crying reaches a peak at about 6 weeks old). So every day you're getting closer to the time when you can get some more sleep. Live in the moment, as babies do. Forget about what you have to do tomorrow or next week. Take it one day, even one hour, at a time, sister.

43

falling through the Days

$DiARY$

The only thing that really helped me to get a grip on the blues was getting home into an environment with fresh air, and the chance to sit outside even if I felt like a zombie and was not at all sure what to do with a tiny baby. It was kind of comforting having the hospital nurses nearby, but nothing like being at home. Besides, I could always call them.

I was so tired in those early days I thought it would never end. I cried toward the end of every day when fatigue started to overwhelm me. We discouraged visitors because rather than offering help, so many seemed to need attention. The visitors who were really helpful were the ones who would pick up the baby or otherwise make themselves useful around the house.

Aunt Peg has forgotten about tiny babies. I remember that Peg didn't get hold of me until I was 3 months old, when Mom died—so she's lost with such a small bundle as Eddy and convinced that every sniffle means malaria, crib death, or convulsions.

All at once I felt lonely, but too tired to make the effort to reach out to friends. It seemed like I was living in a fog of fatigue, robotically waking, feeding the baby, and trying to sleep again, like some kind of demented wet nurse on Valium. Beck told Matt to make me go outside for a walk in the afternoons so at least I would feel like I knew which was day and which was night, and that there was an outside world. This helped a lot.

Eddy was sleeping in the carriage every night because he seemed so TINY in the crib—until this morning when Matt goes in to see him and this weeny, supposedly immobile baby has wiggled his way to the top end of the carriage and is inches away from sticking his head down into a dangerous gap. This gives us a big shock, so we drive to a baby equipment store and get a cradle on rockers. This is the most brilliant decision we've made and we can rock him to sleep. They had these cradles in the nursery for preemie babies.

Every time I think about how I told everyone I'd start work part-time in 8 weeks, I'm overwhelmed with stress and anxiety. I've got to try to go with the flow. Eddy is waking up every 4 hours, which is not too bad compared with some babies, but I am still absolutely exhausted from lack of sleep. Not only do you have to live day by day, but sometimes hour by hour, without looking forward or back.

Marg described the first few weeks as "falling through the day," and she had her sister and mother to help. Matt and I don't have any help, but at least there are two of us. Even so we're lucky if one of us has had a shower by nightfall and somebody can make the dinner. For a while there the washing machine and dryer seemed to be going all day long and there were mountains of diapers . . .

Why didn't I think of it before! We've swapped to disposable diapers and are using the cloth ones as essential, all-purpose shoulder drapes, wipes, bottom cleaners, and soft folded surfaces for the change table. Eddy sleeps up to an extra hour or 2 at night with a disposable diaper on, and I decide he might as well be more comfortable in the daytime as well.

There is a certain guilt in this, and we expect to be raided by the Baby Police or the Environment Squad at any moment. I listen to a caller who calls up a radio station and says that women who use formula and disposable diapers are "lazy." About 100 people call and say they'd like to kill her. Hurrah! I do feel guilty about the environment, so I've joined Greenpeace in Eddy's name.

Breastfeeding is easier than it was at the beginning, but Eddy still has a lot of trouble attaching, especially to the left nipple (which is odd because it has always been his father's favorite). The scar and pain from the cesarean make everything harder, including finding a good position for breastfeeding. I need two pillows to balance him on, and how to feed him insouciantly and— arrgghhh—in public is a complete mystery to me.

His gas is still bad and he cries and cries inconsolably after all the daytime feeds, really screaaaaaaming in the ear of whichever parent is holding him: it's extraordinary how loud a baby can yell. It's so hard not being able to take the pain away, and hard to remain patient with the crying. Yesterday I found myself raising my voice in frustration and saying angrily, "Shut up!" which is about as useful as saying, "Act your age," and as soothing as a lovely death-metal song. Luckily I got hold of myself, stopped raising my voice, and just ended up crying as well. I read Robin Barker's small book called *Crying* over and over, and what the other books say about it as well. But nothing really helps. I just have to keep saying, "This will end, this will end."

I call my doctor's office and ask, "How do I tell, when the baby cries 3 hours after a feeding, whether he's hungry or there's something else wrong?"

"Just feed him when he cries," the receptionist says.

"But it may be too soon and he isn't hungry," I reply, knowing full well from experience that if I feed Eddy after 2 hours he'll projectile vomit. Which, by the way, is such an extremely shocking moment it makes you draw your breath in and open your eyes really wide like an English pantomime actor called Dame Chortlepants.

"Some women feed their babies every hour," she says.

"But how do they do that without going crazy?" I ask.

"Oh," she says airily, "they just do."

How very marvelous.

I'm supposed to be doing all these exercises to help the post-cesarean body, but I might as well be told to read a couple of novels a day—there is just no time at all. And when there is, I'm afraid I need to be horizontal, usually with ear plugs in, my head under the pillow, an eye mask on, dreaming of getting stuck into a bottle of whiskey.

early outings

Baby excursions in the first few weeks can be a tad grueling, and you should never feel you have to go anywhere. It's good just to take your time at home, gradually getting to know your baby, apart from going for short walks in the fresh air, or sitting in the park.

One of the worst things about the early forays out the front door is that you feel you are giving your first public performances

as a new parent. Heaps of new moms cry with frustration the first few times they try to collapse that
damn new stroller into the car or get off a bus with
a baby AND some shopping bags. After a few days
they can do it backward and upside down in the
dark with one foot. It's just a matter of practice.

If you're still getting the hang of changing
diapers, breastfeeding, and working out why the
hell your baby is crying, going out can be a bit
stressful. Also, the virtually full-time nature of
new-baby care doesn't change just because
you're out. Your baby will still need to feed, be
burped, have their diaper and maybe clothes
changed, be settled down to sleep, feed some
more, sleep—or whatever happens at home—
while you're trying to have a cup of tea, stay
awake, and sound intelligible, or get home before dark.

BaBy BaG

Don't worry: it gets easier every time.

so what's in the bag?

The big bag that all parents haul about with them contains whatever you need to change and feed the baby. Its exact contents alter
as the baby grows older, reaching peak capacity during toddler
years, when it includes all diaper-changing equipment plus
sundry snacks, drinks, security blankets, and can't-leave-the-
house-without-Binky-type toys.

The newborn-baby bag will need to contain:

⊚ diapers (plus covers and pins or snappy fasteners, if you use
cloth)—usually 3–4 depending on how long you plan to be out.

⊚ 1–2 changes of outfit in case the going-out clothes get soiled,
which is more likely if you have cloth diapers.

⊚ a surface to change the diapers on—some bags have a built-in
change pad; if yours doesn't, a blanket with a folded cloth diaper
on top or a waterproof-backed change sheet on the floor works
just as well.

⑥ whatever you use to clean your baby's bottom at change time: a small container of water and washcloths or a packet of baby wipes.

⑥ diaper rash cream, which forms a barrier between pee and skin.

⑥ a few plastic bags to bring dirty diapers and clothes home in—reusing supermarket bags is ideal, but check they're not ripped, and tie a knot or two in them for safety until you use them (then tie them up firmly again) in case another baby or a toddler gets hold of them.

⑥ blankets to wrap the baby in, depending on the weather.

⑥ a sun hat if it's hot, a cap or hat if it's cold.

⑥ a couple of clean cloth diapers to drape over the shoulder of anyone holding the baby as a vomit guard or chin wiper.

⑥ a couple of toys suitable for little babies—because newborn babies see mostly contrasts rather than colors for the first 6 months, black-and-white toys are good, and they also like those plastic rings in a chain that you see dangling on strollers, which drugstores sell.

⑥ bibs if you are already using them.

⑥ bottles of freshly made up but cold formula with protective caps if you are bottle-feeding, kept in an insulated bottle carrier. Better still, take the right measurement of cooled boiled water in a bottle (with a cap on) and add formula from individual packages to it (follow individual package instructions) while you are out, then heat it up. This prevents bacteria forming. Never take bottles of hot formula out and never try to keep them hot. Bottles should be drunk within an hour of being heated. Formula individual packages are more expensive than bulk formula, and check the instructions because you may have to make up a larger amount than your baby usually drinks.

Special hint: even if you prefer cloth diapers and a water wash at home, you may find it more convenient to use disposable diapers and commercial baby wipes for excursions.

The main thing about the big bag is this: have it packed and ready to go at all times. Getting around sleeping, feeding, and changing times and actually out of the house is a finely tuned exercise in time management. There is no time for delay while you hunt about looking for things to put in the bag. The exception to this of course is if you are bottle-feeding, in which case you need to take freshly prepared bottles in an insulated bottle carrier.

To have the bag ready, you need duplicates of diaper change lotion, or wipes and barrier cream—probably in smaller, more portable-sized containers or packages than you would buy for use at home. You also need to remember to restock the bag when you get home from an outing. Get used to bringing it in every single time in case the car goes away with it or you need to restock before you go out in the car again.

As well as the big bag, you may need somewhere portable for the baby to sleep. You can take a bassinet (the body of some carriages converts to a basket, which is handy for visiting), or a quilted baby bag, or a lambswool, or a woven baby basket. You can let the baby sleep in the portable infant car seat or carriage if you keep an eye on it all the time. If you set the baby up on the floor, don't forget to draw everyone's attention to this, so the baby doesn't get trodden or sat on. If it's a short visit, newborn babies can be just as comfortable sleeping in their parents' arms as anywhere. Be very aware of other people's toddlers and pets as a potential danger: they may not be used to babies or take any notice of warnings.

You can wear your baby in a pouch as a charming fashion accessory, with optional vomiting feature, as long as the baby is not going to be in a smoky environment, and someone can help you when the baby gets too heavy.

Leaving the house gets easier when feeding and sleeping turn into something resembling a routine. About when they're asking for their first pocket money, maybe.

IMMUNIZATION

Legal requirements for childhood immunizations vary by state. The U.S. has very low rates of infectious diseases, and medical authorities say that to maintain this all kids should be immunized. All child-care centers and schools ask to see children's immunization records or Certificate of Immunization Status (CIS) when they enroll and require that your child be immunized according to your state's law. If there is a medical, personal, or religious reason for not fully immunizing your child, you must obtain a signature from your child's doctor on the certificate noting this exemption.

Some children will still get the diseases they've been immunized against, but the risk is far less after immunization.

Ask about any new vaccines with fewer side effects. (It's appalling, but you may have to pay extra for these.) You can get vaccinations from your child's doctor or a local health clinic. There are routine vaccinations for diphtheria, whooping cough, polio, measles, mumps, rubella, hepatitis B, tetanus, pneumococcal disease, varicella, and *Haemophilus influenzae* type b (Hib). Sometimes three are given in one injection.

Common side effects following immunization are minor fever, soreness where an injection has been given, nausea, and irritability. These should not be too severe or last for very long. Some of the newer vaccines are showing far fewer side effects. Some very rare side effects of vaccines can include convulsions, brain damage, and death, and anti-vaccination activists point to these as unacceptable risks. Another view is often held by those of the older generation who remember the days before vaccinations when thousands of babies died from whooping cough or measles, and several kids in each school had polio and started wearing the braces and using the canes they'd need forever.

Immunization schedule Check with your doctor or American Academy of Pediatrics for your schedule. Sometimes they adjust the recommended schedules, so keep in touch with your doctor or pediatrician as your child grows. Usually there are injections (or sometimes oral vaccines), including vital booster shots, scheduled for when the child is 2 months old, 4 months, 6 months, 1 year, 18 months, 2 years, and 4 years, with a final top-off of some things during the pre-teen and adolescent years before they leave school.

Helping your baby through it Also find out from your doctor what side effects to look out for after the injections, and check that it's safe to give infant Tylenol about 15 minutes before the injection and, in case of a raised temperature, afterwards (98.6° Fahrenheit is normal). Make sure you ask your nurse or doctor the best way for you to take your baby's temperature.

  See Immunization in Help.

and by the way . . .

⑥ Say it loud and say it proud: IF THE CHOICE IS BETWEEN SLEEPING AND THE HOUSEWORK, SLEEP.

⑥ If a certain book or person is making you feel guilty, avoid them. (I burnt Penelope Leach's book in the backyard when I read in it that a "clever" mother shouldn't have to get up more than once a night if she juggles the times of feeds and anticipates her baby's crying at night. You may think it feels bad and wicked to burn a book. It felt FANTASTIC.)

⑥ After a few weeks your boobs will stop being so hard and full before each feeding and stay much floppier, but they are actually producing more and more milk for your growing baby. Don't assume you're running out because your breasts are softer between feedings: your body's just getting more efficient. And it's common for one breast to produce more milk than the other—or be easier for the baby to "draw on."

◎ If you have committed yourself to other projects and you find that looking after a baby is harder than you thought, try to get out of everything you can, if you can, without damaging your work prospects, or decide which prospects you're prepared to sacrifice. Or find ways to get more help with the baby.

◎ Show friends and family how they can help. Many people, not only guys, will be feeling inexperienced and tentative, and scared of hurting a small baby. Show them the way, and everyone will have a better time.

◎ If your baby screams blue murder when you do the bath thing, avoid the stress. It can be much more restful to get in the big bath together and cuddle while you wash, or to just wash bits of your baby with a washcloth. And you don't have to do it every day.

SUDDEN INFANT DEATH SYNDROME (CRIB DEATH)

The cause of SIDS is not known. Basically what happens is that the baby stops breathing. Eighty percent of SIDS deaths happen in the first 6 months. SIDS is now far less common. There is continuing research and a general agreement on how to lower the risk.

1. Sleep your baby on its back, never the tummy. Newborn babies who tend to vomit can be firmly propped on their side with some rolled-up hand towels on either side, or tucked in firmly with a blanket, so that they can't roll onto their back. Ask the hospital nurses to show you, if you're unsure. Roll the baby's head to the side if that is comfortable.

2. Don't smoke when you're pregnant or during your baby's first year, or allow anyone to smoke in the house or the car where the baby is.

3. Don't cover your baby's head when they're sleeping or have soft or puffy toys, bumpers, or bedding such as duvets and pillows in the crib or bassinet, which could cover a tiny head while sleeping.

4. Don't overdress the baby, especially during warm weather.

After about the age of 6 months, babies may stop sleeping in exactly the position you place them in and put themselves into all sorts of positions (bottom up in the air is a particularly entertaining one). Some older babies roll onto their tummies during sleep, and by this age they should be able to move themselves if they get into any breathing trouble.

A few younger babies who are always placed in the same position to sleep may develop a flattened or unusual head shape. In most cases this does no harm and "fixes itself" before school starts. Current SIDS research still indicates babies should be put to sleep on their backs, but you can change the head positions for each sleep, from face turned to one side, then to the other, then to looking straight up. (If your baby always seems to turn its head to face out into the room, you can alternate putting the baby at different ends of the crib, so their head isn't always in the one position.) And if your baby's head seems to be oddly shaped or crooked, have it checked out by a pediatrician for your peace of mind.

 The SIDS Alliance has more detailed advice (see Grief and Loss in Help).

BABY-CARE BOOKS

What to Expect the First Year by Arlene Eisenberg, Heidi E. Murkoff, and Sandee E. Hathaway, Workman Publishing Company, 1989.

The trio is back again with the sequel to *What to Expect When You're Expecting*. A month-to-month guide that's easy to quickly check as the baby grows. One to keep and read when you need to, if you're worried about anything. And when you're finished with it, you can use it as a doorstop: it's a whopper.

The New Parent: The Essential Guide for All First-Time Mothers and Fathers by Miriam Stoppard, DK Publishing, New York, 1998.

Beautifully laid out, with a double-page spread for each theme, the book covers many aspects of pregnancy and then gets onto the business of the baby arriving, baby's first day, what happens to the mother's body after birth, how to look after a baby in the first weeks. Info on breastfeeding and bottle-feeding, and how to put on a diaper, bathe, and dress the bub is well illustrated and short and simple, but this book isn't much good to you if things don't go according to plan. There's a handy section on how the average baby develops at each stage.

The Baby Book: Everything You Need to Know about Your Baby from Birth to Age Two by William and Martha Sears, Little Brown & Co., New York, 2003.

Attachment parenting gurus give their reassuring lowdown on everything from sleeping and crying to feeding, with lots of practical help.

The Fussy Baby Book: Parenting Your High-Need Child from Birth to Age Five by William and Martha Sears, Little Brown & Co., New York, 1996.

For parents who need a hand (and who doesn't!) with a very alert baby, or one who cries a lot, or a toddler fighting for independence. Soothing for babies, and adults!

American Academy of Pediatrics Guide to Your Child's Symptoms
by Donald Schiff, Steven P. Shaw, and American Academy of Pediatrics, Villard Books, New York, 1997.

Organized by children's ages, this resource covers symptoms common to babies through adolescents.

A Parent's Guide to Medical Emergencies by Janet Zand, Rachel Walton, and Bob Rountree, Avery Penguin Putnam, New York, 1997.

Covers basic safety guidelines, CPR for infants and children, and discussion of the most common emergency situations.

For specific books on sleeping and crying see the relevant entries in Help.

forever
after...
(diary)

A number of months down the track I look back at those first weeks and wonder how anyone does it without going completely crazy. Before I had Eddy, when people used to talk about "lack of sleep" I thought of it as an inconvenience—like staying up too late and having a bit of a hangover. Now I can see why they use sleep deprivation as a method of torture. Good old Ed is finally sleeping for 8 hours straight a night.

"We got a good one, la la la," sings Matt.

I can't remember a thing about being pregnant but I still look about 6 months "gone." You know how they say you automatically lose weight when you breastfeed? Nope. And you know how they say you'll lose it when you stop breastfeeding, instead? Not me. Took me about 9 months to feel robust again after the cesarean.

I breastfed for 3 months, then my endometriosis problem started again, and I had to go on the Pill. And the Pill goes through into breast milk and I didn't want to expose Ed to the hormones. Sadly, he no longer regards my boobs as something special, but don't get between him and a bottle of formula. He loves the stuff, and he's thriving on it. He also likes to "chew" rice cereal, severely distressed parsnip, and the tags on all his soft toys.

Some friends have disappeared over the horizon, but I've made new ones at "sleep school" (where we learned what a routine was) and among other moms. Thank God for the childless pals who still call and ask me out. I've hired someone to come and look after Eddy when I'm working part-time from home. Eddy chats away happily in baby language to himself and everyone else, and we've weathered our first ear infection (which crept up and smacked us upside the head while we were waiting for the much-warned-about teething that happened later than most people expect). I'm afraid gummy old Ed is a little backward in the teeth department. At least he's a gifted vomiter or we couldn't hold up our heads at play-group. (And he's a champion drooler, I'll have you know.)

Sometimes I just want to stop the clock and have a week off. Sometimes it's fascinating, sometimes it's dead boring. Sometimes I yearn for a few hours just to myself and yet sometimes it's so lonely. And then there's that moment when he smiles and laughs and reaches out for a cuddle and I think it's the most gorgeous feeling I've ever had.

I suppose the next thing I know Eddy'll be crawling, and going to school, and designing a titanium spaceship, or cooking a dinner party for six. But until then there's a lot of cardboard books about duckies to be read, a lot of ludicrous baby hats to be worn, a lot of walks in the park to be had, and a lot of hurtling round the back-yard being a fairy-seeking missile. And there's a little indent on the back of his neck that's just perfect for kissing, and if you whisper "Oofty Goofty" in his ear he might giggle again. So.
If you'll excuse me . . .

The End. (And just the beginning . . .)

HeLP

BABY HEALTH PROBLEMS

Many babies are born with health problems, ranging from a routine, temporary problem to a serious and dangerous one requiring intensive care and very hard decisions.

You will be able to derive some comfort from knowing that the United States has some of the best-trained and most-dedicated nurses, doctors, pediatricians, specialists, social workers, and counselors in the world. Keep pushing until you feel satisfied that everything that needs to be done is being done, and vote for and put pressure on people whom you believe put medical care as a high priority.

If your baby has a problem, take notes or bring a friend to take notes of your conversations with doctors and other relevant people—it can be a time when shock causes everything to go in one ear and out the other.

There are always parent support groups for specific conditions such as Down's syndrome or spina bifida. You can find them through your pediatrician, your hospital, or the Internet.

American Academy of Pediatrics
Its website has a wealth of information on medical conditions of children from birth to age 21, including an array of articles on birth defects and other congenital conditions.

website: www.aap.org

Association for Retarded Citizens of the Unites States (ARC)
Provides information on cognitive, intellectual, and developmental disabilities.

301-565-3872
email: info@thearc.org
website: www.thearc.org

Federation for Children with Special Needs
Provides support and information to parents of children with disabilities.

617-236-7210
email: fcsninfo@fcsn.org
website: www.fcsn.org

March of Dimes

Contact for information on birth defects, genetics, and prenatal care.

888-663-4637
website: www.modimes.org

Spina Bifida Association of America

800-621-3141

BODY IMAGE

Pregnancy changes a body. You may find these changes confronting or worry about not losing the weight after the baby has arrived. If body image is making you depressed or confused, try one of these books or websites.

www.ifnotdieting.com.au

Bodyiimage expert Dr. Rick Kausman's website is useful for people who feel they eat too much or too little, anyone who feels that thoughts about food are controlling them instead of the other way around. It presents ways you can stop making food the enemy, a study about why diets don't help, and hints for how families can encourage healthy eating and exercise; and there's a lot of smart chat about finding your very own "comfortable weight."

www.about-face.org

This groovy website has a "hall of shame" of advertisers who present ludicrous images of prepubescent body types as something women could or should aim for, and the site contains lots of useful facts about how to fight back against the fashion industry's thin obsession. There are recommended books and Web links about body-image pressures.

www.adiosbarbie.com

This site has a rather amusing feature called "Feed the Supermodel" plus serious help in the form of articles about what to do about your body-image problems.

If Not Dieting, Then What? by Dr. Rick Kausman, Allen and Unwin, Sydney, Australia, 1998.

Dr. Kausman's website is www.ifnotdieting.com.au.

Real Gorgeous: The Truth about Body and Beauty by Kaz Cooke, W.W. Norton and Company, New York, 1996.

My book about how to make friends with your body.

BREASTFEEDING

Nursing Mothers Counsel

A nonprofit organization that provides breastfeeding information and support. They run a 24-hour hotline staffed by volunteer moms who can answer questions about breastfeeding.

408-291-8008
website: www.nursingmothers.org

La Leche League International

An international breastfeeding support group.

847-519-7730
email: lllhq@llli.org
website: www.lalecheleague.org

The Breastfeeding Book by Martha Sears, R.N., and Williams Sears, M.D., Little Brown and Company, New York, 2000.

A comprehensive how-to book by the "attachment-parenting gurus." From starting out to how to wean, it's a useful handbook.

The Breastfeeding Answer Book (Third Edition) by Nancy Mohrbacher and Julie Stock, La Leche League International, Schaumborg, Ill., 1997.

One of the best-selling breastfeeding books on the market, it offers a blend of academic knowledge, clinical expertise, and practical examples.

The New Bestfeeding: Getting Breastfeeding Right for You by Mary Renfrew, Chloe Fisher, and Suzanne Arms, Celestial Arts, Berkeley, Calif., 2000.

Everything you ever wanted to know about breastfeeding, with useful photos and hints (but an unfortunate textbook style).

⊚ For private lactation consultants and renting breast pumps, look under "breast-feeding information and supplies" in the yellow pages.

Bottle Feeding
For bottle feeding, see your pharmacist or pediatrician. Strictly follow the instructions and dosages given by the manufacturers of baby formula. A customer service phone number should be on the can.

CONTRACEPTION AND ABORTION

Surgical abortion is available up to a certain stage of pregnancy, usually in the first trimester, but up to 14 weeks. After 24 weeks abortions are performed only if there are serious health reasons. Contact Planned Parenthood (1-800-230-PLAN) or the National Abortion Federation (1-800-772-9100) for more information. Up to 9 weeks of pregnancy, your doctor can give you two medications that will cause a "miscarriage." You will need to go to a clinic or your doctor's office for the medications.

There is also the option of emergency contraception (the misnamed "morning-after pill") within 120 hours of unprotected sex. You take prescribed pills, wait 12 hours and take some more pills, according to instructions. This means that if an egg has been fertilized, it will not implant in your uterus—in effect, the pregnancy will not have started. If for some reason your doctor is unwilling to prescribe what you need, go to another one, or a family-planning clinic like Planned Parenthood.

CRYING

If your child's crying is driving you crazy, don't just try to put up with it. Learn more about the reasons why your baby cries and contact the following organizations for support.

⊚ Call any of the parent helplines under Parent Services, page 441.

Child Abuse Prevention Services (CAPS)
Offers support and advice to parents and caregivers.

    516-621-0552
    email: caps4kids@aol.com
    website: www.kidsafe-caps.org

National Committee to Prevent Child Abuse
Childhelp U.S.A.
24-hour crisis hotline that offers support
and telephone counseling for parents.

    800-4-A-CHILD

⑥ Parenting websites have many reassuring hints on crying. Look
under World Wide Web and Magazines on page 451.

colichelp.com
A website that offers support and message boards for parents dealing
with colicky babies.

EXERCISE

Fit Pregnancy
A magazine and website that explore healthy exercise during pregnancy.
(Don't worry, nobody really looks like the models do in those pictures!
Or we would have to do away with them by evil and immediate means.)

    website: www.fitpregnancy.com

www.lifematters.com/medicalinfo.html
A website that explains precautions to take while exercising when
pregnant.

Denise Austin's Ultimate Pregnancy Book by Denise Austin, Simon and
Shuster, New York, 1999.

    Fitness guru, Denise Austin's guide to exercise during pregnancy. (If
    you don't feel as perky as Denise, lie on the couch and throw
    popcorn at one of her videos.)

Yoga for Pregnancy by Roslind Widdowson, Creative Publishers,
Minnetonka, Minn., 2001.

    Outlines safe yoga practice during pregnancy. Yoga in pregnancy is
    always easier for people who were already doing it before they
    became pregnant. So if you don't have experience—go especially
    slowly and gently.

FAMILY PLANNING CLINICS

Planned Parenthood

Provides medical advice, treatment, and counseling on a range of issues such as sexually transmitted diseases, contraception, pregnancy care, and abortion. There are clinics all over the country: call for details of your nearest center.

New York
434 West 33rd Street
New York, NY 10001
212-541-7800
email: communications@ppfa.org
website: www.plannedparenthood.com

Chicago
1 Oakbrook Terrace #808
Oakbrook Terrace, IL 60181
630-627-9270

San Francisco
801 Montgomery Street, Fifth Floor
San Francisco, CA 94133
415-956-8856

Washington, D.C.
1780 Massachusetts Avenue, NW
Washington, D.C. 20036
202-785-3351

GRIEF AND LOSS

It is rare, but some babies die in the last weeks of pregnancy and are induced stillborn. Some babies die soon after birth or in the following weeks. Often the general baby books are no help to grieving parents, and often you can't remember what you've been told by medical staff because of the shock and grief. During these terrible times there are lots of experts who may be able to offer you a great deal of help:

- midwives, nurses, and doctors
- hospital social workers
- counselors or therapists
- the SIDS Alliance, if relevant

A friend or relative who can help you to take notes of what is said by these people about your options can be invaluable. Your head may be spinning trying to take in too much new information.

There are support groups for parents and siblings affected by the death of a baby, or for those trying to deal with a baby who has special needs. Ask your hospital or pediatrician to put you in touch with them.

People react very differently to grief—some don't want to talk about it, and this can seem to others who grieve differently that they do not care as much. This is not the case. Grief counselors can help a couple or a whole family, including other children, to understand what has happened. Your hospital or doctor should be able to help you find one who specializes in the loss of a baby (that's important). Or see contacts below.

The Compassionate Friends
A support service for bereaved parents. Contact them to find your local chapter.

> 877-969-0100
> website: www.compassionatefriends.org

SHARE Pregnancy and Infant Loss Support, Inc.
A nondenominational organization providing support to those affected by the death of a baby through early pregnancy loss, stillbirth, or newborn death.

> 800-821-6819 or 636-947-6164
> email: share@nationalshareoffice.com
> website: www.nationalshareoffice.com

The MISS Foundation
Provides emergency support to families in crisis after the death of their baby or young child.

> website: www.misschildren.org

SIDS Alliance
Provides help with grief, as well as information about helping to prevent deaths of babies.

> 410-653-8226
> website: www.sidsalliance.org

Empty Cradle, Broken Heart: Surviving the Death of Your Baby by Deborah Davis, Fulcrum Publishing, Golden, Colo., 1996.

One of the best-selling books on the market about parental loss. It offers reassurance to parents who are dealing with anger, guilt, and sadness. Features a special chapter on how fathers may grieve differently.

Help, Comfort, and Hope after Losing Your Baby in Pregnancy or the First Year by Hannah Lothrop, Fisher Books, Boulder, Colo., 1997.

This book explains the grieving process, and also provides an extensive list of resources for bereaved parents.

IMMUNIZATION

Your doctor should have all immunization schedules to show you what your child will need and provide a Certificate of Immunization Status for your child. The American Academy of Pediatrics also has immunization schedules available.

National Immunization Information Hotline

800-232-2522

Center for Disease Control and Prevention

Contact for information on immunizations and diseases.

website: www.cdc.gov

www.childrensvaccine.org
www.polioeradication.org

Two websites that will tell you what's going on in the underdeveloped world, and about the benefits of immunization.

INFERTILITY

Counselors are available at all infertility and IVF clinics or through any major hospital, which your doctor can refer you to. It's important to go to a counselor specializing in infertility. They can best help you explore your medical options and also put you in touch with a support group.

www.fertilethoughts.com
A website for connecting with other couples who are experiencing infertility. It features a search engine to locate doctors in your area who specialize in infertility treatment.

RESOLVE The National Infertility Association
Offers support and information for couples struggling with infertility.
> 888-623-0744
> website: www.resolve.org

Overcoming Infertility by Robert Jansen, W.H. Freeman, New York, 1998.
> Subtitled "A Compassionate Resource for Getting Pregnant," this is a look at the many different medical and "natural" fertility treatments available, your options, and the emotional aspect of each treatment. Written by a doctor in the field.

Experiencing Infertility by Debby Peoples and Harriett Rovener Ferguson, W.W. Norton, New York, 2000.
> Written by women who have experienced infertility, this book combines medical information with emotional support.

MIDWIVES

American College of Nurse-Midwives
> 202-728-9860
> website: www.acnm.org

Midwives Alliance of North America
> 888-923-6262
> website: www.mana.org

MULTIPLE BIRTHS

Contact the following organizations for counseling and support, and to find your nearest club. You can get advice on feeding and other practical logistics, and swap or buy equipment suitable for a bigger brood.

National Organization of Mothers of Twins Clubs, Inc.

> P.O. Box 23188
> Albuquerque, NM 87192
> 505-275-0955
> website: www.nomotc.org

Triplet Connection

> P.O. Box 99571
> Stockton, CA 95209
> 209-474-0885
> website: www.tripletconnection.org

Twins Magazine

> 5350 South Roslyn Street, Suite 80
> Englewood, CO 80111
> 800-328-3211
> website: www.twinsmagazine.com

The Multiple Pregnancy Sourcebook by Nancy Bowers, R.N., B.S.N., Contemporary Books, Lincolnwood, Ill., 2001.

> Written by a nurse and mother of twins, this book concentrates on a multiple pregnancy and coping in the first weeks after birth: both highs and lows are covered.

Twins! by Connie L. Agnew, M.D., Alan H Klein, M.D., and Jill Alison Ganon, HarperCollins, New York, 1997.

> Similar mainstream approach and format to *What to Expect When You're Expecting*, this also has some advice about the first year with two babies.

Twins, Triplets, and More: Their Nature, Development, and Care by Elizabeth Bryan, St. Martin's Press, New York, 1998.

> The author is a pediatrician who specializes in multiple births.

NATURAL HEALTH CARE

American Massage Therapy Association
Details on safe massage procedures for pregnant women.

> 820 Davis Street, Suite 100
> Evanston, IL 60201-4444
> 847-864-0123
> website: www.amtamassage.org

American Holistic Medical Association

> 505-292-7582
> website: www.holisticmedicine.org

American Association of Oriental Medicine
Lists licensed acupuncture practitioners across the country.

> 888-500-7999
> email: info@aaom.org
> website: www.aaom.org

PARENT GROUPS AND HOTLINES

National Association of Mothers' Centers
Meet other mothers in a supportive place. Share your experiences and learn more about your child's development. Check out the website for a mothers' center near you.

> 64 Division Avenue
> Levittown, NY 11756
> 800-645-3828
> website: www.motherscenter.org

Parents Anonymous
Offers parenting support groups and tips. Check out the website or give them a call to find out about meetings in your area.

> 909-621-6184

Postpartum Support International
Runs support groups across the country for parents.

> 927 North Kellogg Avenue
> Santa Barbara, CA 93111
> 805-967-7636
> website: www.postpartum.net

www.babyzone.com
www.babycenter.com
www.parenting.com
These are some useful parenting websites.

Here are listings for parent and crisis hotlines and family centers by state. These hotlines offer phone counseling and should refer you to support groups, in-person counseling, parenting classes, and other parenting resources in your area.

ALABAMA

CONTACT Helpline
24-hour crisis line.
800-239-1117

ALASKA

Anchorage Center for Families
Parenting education and support, in-home services, and a 24-hour hotline.
907-276-8511

ARIZONA

Parent Information and Referral Center
800-690-2282

Parent Assistance Program Hotline
800-732-8193

ARKANSAS

Jones Center for Families
501-756-8090

CALIFORNIA

Parental Stress Services
24-hour crisis hotline for parents.
888-829-3777

FLORIDA

Parent Help-Line
Provides 24-hour telephone counseling, crisis intervention, information, and referral to services that can help children and parents through difficult times.
813-234-1234

HAWAII

The Parentline
800-816-1222

ILLINOIS

Parent Hotline
For parents who need help with prenatal and newborn care.
800-545-2200 or 888-727-5889

INDIANA

Family Service Association of Monroe County
Offers counseling, parent support, and workshops on child rearing.
812-339-1555

KANSAS

> **Parent Helpline**
> 800-332-6378

KENTUCKY

> **Parent Helpline**
> 24-hour hotline.
> 800-432-9251

> **Health Access; Nuturing Development (HANDS)**
> Offers home visitation services for new parents.
> 502-564-2154

LOUISIANA

> **Parent Helpline**
> 800-348-KIDS

MARYLAND

> **Parent Warmline**
> Offers child-rearing advice.
> 301-929-WARM

MASSACHUSETTS

> **Parent Line**
> 617-421-1789
> **Parental Stress Line**
> 800-632-8188

MICHIGAN

> **Parent Help Line**
> 800-942-4357

MINNESOTA

> **Crisis Connection**
> 612-379-6363

> **Fathers' Crisis Line**
> 612-874-1509

MISSOURI

> **Parental Stress Hotline**
> 800-367-2543

> **ParentLink Warmline**
> 800-367-2543

NEW HAMPSHIRE

Parent Line
800-640-6486

NEW JERSEY

Contact Crisis Line
856-795-2155

NEW MEXICO

Family Crisis Hotline
505-325-1906

NEW YORK

Parent Helpline
800-342-7472

NORTH DAKOTA

Parent Line
800-258-0808

OHIO

Family Link Line
513-946-LINK

OKLAHOMA

Parenting Helpline
877-446-6865

OREGON

Parent Helpline
800-345-5044

PENNSYLVANIA

Parent to Parent of Pennsylvania
800-986-4550

TENNESSEE

Parent Helpline
800-356-6767

TEXAS

Family Forward Texas Parent Heartline
800-554-2323

VERMONT

> **Parents Assistance Line**
> 800-727-3687
>
> **Parents Stress Line**
> 800-244-5373

WASHINGTON

> **Family Help Line**
> 206-233-0156

WEST VIRGINIA

> **Family Matters Hotline**
> 888-983-2645

WISCONSIN

> **Florence County Parenting Warmline**
> Support for the day-to-day challenges of parenting.
> 888-432-6495

CANADA

> **Parent Help Line**
> 24-hour tips and information on child rearing for Canadians.
> 888-603-9100

PARENT SERVICES

Child Help National Hotline
24-hour advice and referrals for parents who have questions or emergencies.

> 800-422-4453

Boys Town National Hotline
Provides crisis intervention, information, and referrals for children (girls and boys) and families. Spanish-speaking counselors are available.

> 800-448-3000

POISON

Poison Control
This 24-hour hotline connects you to the closest poison center.
> 800-222-1222

POSTPARTUM DEPRESSION

See also Parent Groups and Hotlines and Parent Services: most of the organizations listed there can help you. Ask your doctor to refer you to a counselor or center, or you can contact your nearest women's health clinic.

Depression after Delivery
A national lobby and support group offering practical help and advice.
> 888-404-7763
> website: www.ppmdsupport.com

Postpartum Support International
Provides a forum and referral service and has lots of helpful information.
> 805-967-7636
> website: www.postpartum.net

This Isn't What I Expected: Overcoming Postpartum Depression by Karen Kleiman and Valerie Davis Raskin, Bantam Books, New York, 1994.
> A book about how to get back from the badlands. Presents options for treatment and info for male partners. Helps you understand you're not alone and get your confidence back.

PREMATURE BABIES

Ask your obstetrician, midwife, or hospital to put you in touch with a support group if your baby is premature.

American Association of Premature Infants
Offers support to parents of premature babies.

> website: www.aapi-online.org

www.preemie-l.org
The website of a nonprofit parents-of-preemies organization. Answers frequently asked questions, and provides fact sheets and a newsletter.

Caring for Your Premature Baby by Alan H. Klein and Jill Alison Ganon, HarperPerennial, New York, 1998.

> Concentrates on really premature (not preterm) babies (preterm are the subject of one chapter). Includes practical advice, real stories from other parents, and hints on dealing with the medical world. Heavy on breastfeeding advocacy.

SAFETY

The following contacts provide a heap of services such as phone advice, safety products, and printed information including fact sheets on separate safety subjects. Most baby-care books also have lists of things you can do to make a home safe (such as move to another one). (Sorry.)

Child Equipment

Auto Safety Hotline
Has recall information on automobiles and child car seats.
888-327-4236

Consumer Reports
For information on car seats, cribs, and other baby products.
website: www.consumerreports.org

The Danny Foundation
Provides information on crib safety.
800-83-DANNY
website: www.dannyfoundation.org

Safety Belt Safe U.S.A.
Information on car seats.
website: www.carseat.org

U.S. Consumer Product Safety Commission
800-638-2772
website: www.cpsc.gov

Pregnancy Safety

Food and Drug Administration
For up-to-date health information.
888-723-3366

National Healthy Mothers, Healthy Babies Coalition
Information on pregnancy. The national office can connect you to the
Healthy Mothers, Healthy Babies Coalition in your state.
703-836-6110
email: info@hmhb.org
website: www.hmhb.org

National Institute for Occupational Safety and Health (NIOSH)
Info on safety at work for pregnant women.
800-356-4674
website: www.cdc.gov/niosh/homepage.html

Occupational Safety and Health Administration (OSHA)
Governmental organization that has information on safety at your
workplace.
200 Constitution Avenue NW
Washington, D.C. 20210
202-693-1999
website: www.osha.gov

Child-Proofing and Safety

National Safe Kids Campaign
Features a ton of information on baby- and child-proofing your home.
800-441-1888
website: www.safekids.org

Poison Control
24-hour poison hotline.
800-222-1222

SINGLE PARENTS

National Organization of Single Mothers
The HQ can put you in touch with a group in your area, give practical advice, and inform you of your rights and entitlements.

> 704-888-5437
> website: www.singlemothers.org

Single Parents Association
There's probably a single-parenting support group in your area. To find out, phone:

> 800-704-2102

Federal Office of Child Support Enforcement
A government organization that enforces the payment of child support. If you contact the federal office or check out its website you can get contact information for your state's child support enforcement agency.

> Federal Office of Child Support Enforcement
> Administration for Children and Families
> 370 L'Enfant Promenade S.W.
> Washington, D.C. 20201
> website: www.acf.hhs.gov/programs/cse/

SLEEPING

If you're not getting enough sleep, you'll find everything else much more difficult. You may have a baby who won't nap during the day and then is cranky by evening, or one who wakes up often at night, perhaps wanting to be fed every 2 hours, even when a few months old. Many people who find themselves at their wits' end now seek help with such problems from sleep seminars, clinics, or residential (live-in for a few days) programs. Check hospitals near you to see if they have a day-visit or residential sleep program. These can be very expensive and may be only available to those people with health insurance.

◎ There are some other sources of great information and help.

Silent Nights: Overcoming Sleep Problems in Babies and Children by Brian Symon, Oxford University Press, Oxford, U.K., 1999.

Written by a doctor who has made sleep difficulties his specialty. An easy-to-get-into book that identifies lots of sleep problems and possible solutions, ranging from newborns and the first weeks to toddlers and children. Covers special disruptive occasions such as daylight saving time, moving homes, relatives who sabotage your routine, and first nightmares.

Secrets of the Baby Whisperer by Tracy Hogg, Ballantine, New York, 2001.

This sensible, kind, and reassuring book has the inside scoop on how to set up a daily routine to encourage sleep for everyone, how to get a baby to sleep, and the crucial task—how to recognize a baby's tired signs (like the signals from a baseball manager, they can be hard to decode unless you are in the know!).

The Baby Book and **The Fussy Baby Book: Parenting Your High Need Child from Birth to Age Five** by William and Martha Sears, Little and Brown, New York, 2003 and 1996.

Both books have heaps of ideas for settling, soothing, and sanity.

Solve Your Child's Sleep Problems by Dr. Richard Ferber, Simon and Shuster, New York, 1986.

Dr. Ferber is the Big Cheese at the Boston Children's Hospital Center for Pediatric Sleep Disorders and is known as the "controlled crying guy." His thesis includes his views on what children associate with sleep, and how to teach your child to fall asleep on his or her own by letting him or her "cry it out" for increasingly longer amounts of time each night. Also covers nighttime disturbances, the importance of a daily schedule to nighttime sleeping, and how to stop night feeding.

www.babycenter.com
www.babyzone.com
www.mumstheword.com.au
www.parenting.com

These websites have advice on sleeping and crying issues, as well as other baby business.

TEENAGE AND YOUNG MOMS

Being a pregnant teenager has special problems and special advantages. Having a baby is a big challenge if you're not yet fully an adult yourself, and, like any pregnant woman, you need to know that all the services and help you want are available.

Hospitals and clinics should have special information, classes, and support groups for you, and you can find out about them from your doctor, clinic, or social worker. They may help you work out plans for your pregnancy and birth; learn how to look after the baby (or suggest organizations that will teach you) and plan for the future, such as getting back to school or into work; arrange financial help if your family is not being supportive; and deal with any other worries you might have, speak to your parents if that's difficult for you, and even help you find accommodation.

It's really important for you and the baby to eat MORE than usual while you are pregnant. Don't eat less to try to look as if you're not pregnant; it is really dangerous to diet during pregnancy. You need more nutrients and calories (not junk food) than a pregnant woman who's older than you because, while your baby is growing, you're still growing too.

Don't forget that doctors are required by law to keep secret anything you tell them—so if you're afraid of your family finding out, tell your doctor and he or she should put you in contact with a hospital youth worker or someone else who can help. It's important that you get medical care even if your family doesn't know.

Call Planned Parenthood or a women's clinic and ask to be put in contact with a staff member who works with teenage moms. Often, they will have books or videos you can borrow, and well as special clinics and confidential advice. (They will not tell your parents anything if you don't want them to.)

Boston University: Teen Pregnancy and Maternal/Neonatal Health
Features information about your health and the health of your baby during pregnancy and after birth.

> website: www.bu.edu/cohis/teenpreg/preg/healthy.htm

Planned Parenthood
(See Family Planning Clinics on page 431 for complete details.)

> website: www.plannedparenthood.org/teens/index.htm

hipMama

A website and magazine with information on parenting for young mothers.

> P.O. Box 12525
> Portland, OR 97212
> website: www.hipmama.com

WOMEN'S HEALTH CENTERS

About one-third of hospitals across the country have a Women's Health Center, and there are hundreds of private practices specializing in women's health. The following Women's Health Centers are designated by the U.S. government as National Centers of Excellence in Women's Health and are considered some of the best centers in the country that specialize in women's issues ranging from pregnancy to breast cancer to mental illness.

CALIFORNIA

University of California, Los Angeles National Center of Excellence in Women's Health
100 UCLA Medical Plaza Drive, Suite 290
Los Angeles, CA 90095-7075
Clinical services contact: 800-825-2631

University of California, San Francisco National Center of Excellence in Women's Health
2356 Sutter Street, First Floor, Box 1694
San Francisco, CA 94143-1694
Clinical services contact: 415-353-2668

ILLINOIS

University of Illinois at Chicago Center of Excellence in Women's Health
1640 West Roosevelt Road, Room 503
Chicago, IL 60608
Clinical services contact: 800-UIC-1002

INDIANA

Indiana University School of Medicine National Center of Excellence in Women's Health
535 Barnhill Drive, RT-150
Indianapolis, IN 46202
Clinical services contact: 317-630-2243

LOUISIANA

Tulane Xavier National Center of Excellence in Women's Health
Universities of Louisiana
Tulane University School of Public Health and Tropical Medicine
127 Elks Place, EP-7
New Orleans, LA 70112
Clinical services contact: 877-588-5100

MASSACHUSETTS

Boston University Center of Excellence in Women's Health
Boston University Medical Center
720 Harrison Avenue
Doctor's Office Building, Suite 1108
Boston, MA 02118
Clinical services contact: 617-638-7428

Harvard Medical School Women's Hospital
75 Francis Street, Neville 210
Boston, MA 02115
Clinical services contact: 800-417-4423

MICHIGAN

University of Michigan Health System
Department of Obstetrics, Gynecology
1342 Taubman Center (Level One)
1500 East Medical Center Drive, Room L-4000
Ann Arbor, MI 48109-0276
Clinical services contact: 734-936-8886

PENNSYLVANIA

Magee-Womens Hospital University of Pittsburgh
Department of Obstetrics, Gynecology, and Reproductive Sciences
300 Halket Street
Pittsburgh, PA 15213-3180
Clinical services contact: 412-647-4747

Drexel University Institute for Women's Health and Leadership
The Gatehouse
3300 Henry Avenue
Philadelphia, PA 19129
Clinical services contact: 215-842-7007

PUERTO RICO

University of Puerto Rico, The Women and Health Center
Medical Sciences Campus
P.O. Box 365067
San Juan, PR 00936-5067
Clinical services contact: 787-764-3707

WASHINGTON

University of Washington, Women's Health Care Center
4245 Roosevelt Way NE, Third Floor
Campus Box 354765
Seattle, WA 98105
Clinical services contact: 800-826-1121

WISCONSIN

UW Center for Women's Health & Women's Health Research
6W-Meriter, Park
202 South Park Street
Madison, WI 53715
Clinical services contact: 608-267-5566

WORK: GOING BACK

Find out if your company has any programs that might suit you—job sharing or part-time options. Check what this means for benefits such as sick leave and vacation time.

◎ See if your state or federal government offers any subsidies or programs that might help you ease back into the workforce if you've been out of it for a long while. You can also contact the union that covers your work area (if any) and ask if they have any help or programs available.

Child Care Aware
This group can give you a list of licensed child-care centers in your area.
> 800-424-2246
> email: info@childcareaware.org
> website: www.childcareaware.org

Women's Bureau of the U.S. Department of Labor
Information about the rights of pregnant women and women with families.
> 800-827-5335

U.S. Equal Opportunity Commission
> website: www.eeoc.gov

WORLD WIDE WEB AND MAGAZINES

If you have access to the Internet, you can contact heaps of websites about all aspects of pregnancy and parenthood. It's best to use your search engine on a specific topic, rather than getting a huge list of them here, because websites come and go. (Beware of those pesky porn sites that pop up when you're looking for pregnancy information. And avoid any site that seems to be pushing advertisers' products or trying to get your details on a mailing list.) Get consumer information before buying anything online. Websites can vary from large community sites with chatrooms to individual obstetricians' sites with articles about pregnancy.

The Rough Guide to Shopping Online by Paul Simpson, Rough Guides, New York, 2001.
> Good sites, and lots of hints on protecting your money and privacy from cyberpirates.

Useful Websites
www.salonmagazine.com/mwt/index.html
Salon online magazine has a section called "Mothers Who Think," which has articles archived about parenthood and related issues.

www.babycenter.com
A gigantic commercial website with all sorts of articles, advice, and chat room action on subjects from pregnancy (you) to toddling (the kid) and beyond. Sections on sleeping, crying, diapers, almost anything you can

think of. Supported by online sales of kid-related stuff, as are most baby websites.

www.babyzone.com
A pregnancy and parenting website of *Parenting* magazine, this site has an enviable archive of all manner of subjects divided into sections on pregnancy, baby, toddler, and child. Easy to navigate and beautifully presented.

www.parentsoup.com
A minestrone of parenting advice on everything from potty training to step-parenting and poison ivy first aid.

www.americanbaby.com
The website of *American Baby* magazine has everything from a "maternity bra sizer" feature to an "ask the expert" service with an OBGYN and pediatrician.

Magazines

Fit Pregnancy
Full of fitness and nutritional information from the publishers of *Shape* magazine.

Parents
Articles about the daily life and worries of today's moms. With features on a wide range of topics including child care, nutrition, fashion, child development, health, pregnancy, marriage, money matters, schooling, and discipline.

Child
Features information on pregnancy and child rearing.

acknowledgments

U.S. edition: A heartfelt thank you to editor Carrie Rodrigues, designer Betsy Stromberg, and everyone else at Ten Speed Press. And thanks go to Dr. Patty Robertson of UCSF Medical Center and mother and proofreader Karen O'Donnell Stein for their reviews.

Original edition: Thanks are due to many people who went so far out of their way to help with this book they needed a cut lunch and some travel insurance.

The unbelievably fabulous Dr. Maria Dziardek, developmental biologist at the Department of Anatomy and Cell Biology at Melbourne University, almost drowned under a mountain of faxes, and read and corrected an early draft of each and every What's Going On section.

Manuscript readers and fact-checkers included Ruth Trickey of the Clifton Hill Natural Health Centre, who provided constant assistance with medical and herbal matters; Melanie Pitts, midwife and childbirth educator from Masada Hospital, Melbourne; and Dr. Ann Olsson, obstetrician and gynecologist, Adelaide, who made many useful suggestions. Independent midwife Annie Sprague answered almost endless queries.

I couldn't be more grateful to Dr. Len Kliman, obstetrician and gynaecologist, to whom I entrusted my life and my baby's life, and the first draft of the manuscript. We were all in safe hands.

Research for all the special topics was meticulously compiled originally by Fiona Wood, with some assistance from Aimee Said.

Without exception, staff from the Royal Women's Hospital in Melbourne who were approached gave immediate and remarkably generous help with reading bits of the manuscript, checking facts or providing information. Dietitian Elizabeth Gasparini from the Department of Nutrition and Dietetics contributed to and checked relevant parts of the manuscript, as did Sue Fawcett, an associate genetic counselor from the Genetic Counseling Service. Thanks also to Kay Oke, an infertility counselor in the Reproductive Biology Unit, and Kym Davey from the Young Mothers' Clinic.

Thanks are also due to Dr. Mike Paech, specialist anesthetist at the King Edward Memorial Hospital for Women, in Perth, for his information on pain relief during labor and delivery; Deb Withers and Jo Durst from the SIDS Research Foundation; Michelle Mason from the Masada Hospital Day Stay Program for Mothers and Babies in Melbourne; the Monash Medical Centre IVF program's Professor David de Kretzer, who

ACKNOWLEDGMENTS ◎ 4 5 5

discussed with me how long people should "try" before seeking help; Dr Tony Holmes, director of the Craniofacial Unit at the Royal Children's Hospital in Melbourne, and Dr David David, head of the Australian Craniofacial Unit in Adelaide, for advising on baby head shapes and sleeping positions; and Dr. Henrietta Williams of the Family Planning Association. Independent lactation consultant Margaret Callaghan gave the bosom bits a once-over.

For help with the bibliography and the generous donation of pregnancy and baby books to the Young Mothers' Clinic at the Royal Women's Hospital, thanks to J. G., Imogen Cook and Gab Connellan at Penguin Books, the publicity staff at Random House, Catherine Proctor of Pan Macmillan, Roberta Marcroft at HarperCollins, Michelle Hurley at Allen and Unwin, Stephanie van den Broek and Nicki Robilliard at Dorling Kindersley, Dimity Barber at Oxford University Press, Fiona Robinson at Simon and Schuster, and Rosey Cummings at Tweddle Child and Family Health Service.

I never understood why authors bang on about how their editor did so much work and saved them from making terrible mistakes. Oo-er. Now I get it. Thank you Lesley Dunt.

Thanks as well to Sandy Cull and Leonie Stott for their collaboration and hard work on the design. And a very big hurrah to the Executive Publisher at Penguin Books, Julie Gibbs—every author should have one.

I'd like to thank also all the Lorraines, especially Jane Drury and Katie Purvis for their proofreading and editorial help, and Sandra Jackson.

The largest thanks of all must go to the remarkable Geoffrey Leonard.

By its nature this book is subjective, as well as including about a gerzillion facts. Those acknowledged here are not responsible for errors, or for current fashionable advice and accepted statistics that may change in an inkling. Nor are they responsible for any of the author's own, damned flighty opinions.

And just one final point. When authors compare producing a book to having a baby, they need a damned good slapping.

index

we'd love to hear from you

Please write to us about:

⑥ your experiences of any aspect of pregnancy, birth and the first few weeks of caring for your newborn baby

⑥ anything covered in the book that you'd like to comment on or share your feelings about.

You can send a letter, postcard or even a photocopy of the Your Record sections you've filled in. Please include your name, age and town, and write to:

Kaz Cooke
c/o Ten Speed Press
P.O. Box 7123
Berkeley, CA
94707
U.S.A.

Kaz Cooke is an illustrator, and mom from Australia, where the first edition of this book is still a best-seller. She does not divide her time between a New York loft, a Tuscan farmhouse, and the Florida beachfront, and she didn't really call her baby Oofty Goofty. What's more, there appears to be some mashed banana in her hair.